the
Hedge People

how I kept my sanity and sense
of humor as an alzheimer's caregiver

Louise Carey

Keep smiling at life!
Louise Carey

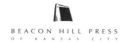

BEACON HILL PRESS
OF KANSAS CITY

ISBN 978-0-8341-2468-4

Printed in the United States of America

Cover Design: Arthur Cherry
Interior Design: Sharon Page

Library of Congress Cataloging-in-Publication Data

Carey, Louise, 1952-
    The hedge people : how I kept my sanity and sense of humor as an Alzheimer's caregiver /
Louise Carey.
        p. cm.
    ISBN 978-0-8341-2468-4 (pbk.)
    1. Caregivers—Prayers and devotions. 2. Caring—Religious aspects—Christianity. 3.
Dementia—Patients—Care. I. Title.
    BV4910.9.C37 2009
    242'.88—dc22

                                                                            2009023042

10 9 8 7 6 5 4 3 2

Contents

Introduction   5

  1. The Hedge People   7

  2. The Mystery Woman   12

  3. A Cloth of All Trades   16

  4. The Mysterious Duo   20

  5. The Train from Long Beach   25

  6. Nighttime Woes   30

  7. The Novel   36

  8. The Radio Program   42

  9. My Neighbor   46

10. The "Don'tist"   51

11. Locked In, Locked Out   57

12. A Tenacious Little Dog   62

13. Choir Practice   65

14. The Edge of the Pool   72

15. The Activity Director   78

16. The Spirit Is Fine   83

17. The Juggler   88

18. Something Seems Suspicious   93

19. The Sweepstakes   98

20. Home Alone   105

21. It Seemed So Harmless   110

22. Getting It All Together   114

23. A Calculated Risk   117

24. The Final Launch   121

Epilogue   127

Introduction

My father-in-law, Art, came to live with us in his ninety-fourth year of life and his eighth year of dementia. He lived with us until he passed away two years and three months later.

A few months after his arrival, I happened to meet a friend in the grocery store. She is older and more affluent than I. We were merely acquaintances until her husband was diagnosed with Alzheimer's disease and Art came to live with us. Now we have a common bond that has forged a strong friendship.

That morning in the grocery store, we shared a bit about how our day was going. Her husband was focused on hurricanes. He had been watching CNN, and all he could talk about was hurricanes. When I told her that I had listened to Art read the address label on his *Reader's Digest* at least twenty times that morning, she got a knowing smile on her face—the smile of a comrade who truly understood.

"I read a quote this morning," she said. "It was *If you smile at life, life will smile back at you.* Let's keep smiling at life."

The goal of this book is to encourage caregivers of patients with dementia to keep smiling at life. Caring for a person with Alzheimer's disease or other forms of dementia is terribly frustrating. Mixed with the frustration is a deep sadness caused by the loss of the person we used to know and a haunting fear of what is to come. *The Hedge People* gives caregivers an opportunity to laugh about the situations we experienced due to Art's dementia and hopefully will enable them to start seeing the humor in their own daily challenges.

The stories in this book are true. When Art came to live with us, my sister-in-law said, "Louise, look for the 'merry heart' moments, and e-mail them to me." Her request was a gift of sunshine to me. It encouraged me to look for and share the unique and humorous things that happened. My purpose in sharing these stories with other caregivers is to shed a different light on the daily drudgeries of caregiving—and to offer the reader permission to "keep smiling at life"!

1 ✳ The Hedge People

We have a large front yard surrounded by a tall cypress hedge. Let me clarify that—it's a hedge to everyone except Art. When Art looks out into our yard, he sees the hedge not as a hedge but as a group of people. The trunks of the hedge look like legs to his failing eyesight, and in his mind there's a large group of people out there. I call them "the hedge people."

The hedge people seem to draw Art. Having been a pastor who started fledgling churches, Art sees any group of people as a potential congregation.

The first time he spotted the hedge people, he whispered in awe, "There's a small part of a million people out there. Do you think any of them play the piano?"

"Not a one," I answered, quite sure I was being truthful.

Sometimes Art stands on the front steps and preaches to the hedge people. On other occasions he goes out to talk to them personally. I have watched him march determinedly down the sidewalk, only to arrive at the hedge and look around, bewildered. Where did they go? All those people were just here, and now not a one is in sight.

Not long ago, Art had the notion that he was a delegate at the Brethren National Conference. He searched frantically for pen and paper. He needed to hurry because he did not want to miss the missionary reports. After I had equipped him with the necessary supplies, he headed out to join the hedge people for the session. It was not long before he came back in the house, discouraged. He could not find the meeting.

"Oh, I heard that the missionary reports will be at 5 P.M.— you have time to take a nap," I suggested.

He was relieved that there was time to rest with such a demanding schedule. "I'm getting old, you know," he confided.

There are times the hedge people get hungry and need to be fed. One day Art searched long and hard for Leah Belle, his deceased wife. She was hiding out. That woman—trying to get out of work when there were so many hungry people to feed!

By noon, Art himself was getting hungry. He gazed out the window and exclaimed, "There are at least seventy-five people out there, and they've been standing in line for hours. Not one of them has gotten a plate. I'm not getting in that line."

"Why don't you come back here in the kitchen? I'll give you a plate right now," I offered.

He happily sat down at the breakfast nook. What a lucky break! He could eat right away without standing in line with the hedge people.

One chilly morning Art was on a mission. He was insistent that the hedge people needed to come inside. They were getting cold, and he was worried about them.

"They need to get out of that 'outfit'"—his all-purpose, generic word for any noun that eluded him—"and come in where it's warm," he said.

He stood on the front step, calling and waving them in.

Harmless activity, I thought and went back to the office to get some work done.

Pretty soon Art found me. He needed my help.

"Why?" I asked.

"Us," he replied.

"Us?"

"Yes, I thought if we did it together, they'd find it more interesting."

"I have about ten more minutes of work, and then I can come," I told him, hoping that in the meantime he would forget.

Undaunted, Art hurried off to try again. In a flash he returned. "They won't come for a guy, but they'd come running for a girl," he said hopefully.

I went out to the front porch with Art at my side and called in a stage whisper, "Come in! Come in!"

Art was sure that my location and technique were not adequate for the task. We had to get closer, call louder, and make swooping motions with our arms. Taking me by the hand, he tromped determinedly to the middle of the front lawn and demonstrated how to do it.

Then he looked at me expectantly. It was time for me to join in. So there we stood, in the middle of the front yard, waving our arms and loudly beckoning the hedge people to take refuge from the cold.

My mind was racing. *Could the neighbors see us through the hedge? No doubt they could hear us! What in the world would they think?*

At best, they would think that we were doing some morning calisthenics. At worst, they would be sadly shaking their heads and saying, "It's been too much for her. She's lost her mind."

Oblivious to my discomfort, Art was in high spirits. It's a lonely task ministering to hedge people. But today he had help!

We called loud and long, "Come in! Come in! It's cold! Come in!"

In spite of our enthusiastic gesturing and calling, those hedge people were impossible to convince. Finally I stopped and looked at Art. "They're not coming. Why don't we go inside and have a cup of coffee? We can regroup and try again later."

Dementia was on my side. Somewhere in that cup of coffee, Art forgot all about the hedge people shivering in the cold. I had a little more trouble putting them out of my mind. It's one thing to be a casual observer of Art's ministry to the hedge people, but it was another thing altogether to become an active participant.

Caregiver's Prayer

Dear God, I accept this job of caregiving as your will for me right now. Help me think of the past with thankfulness rather than a sense of loss. Give me peace and joy as I accept today for what it is, and protect me from longing for what it might have been.

Just Between Caregivers
The Call to Caregiving

During my lifetime, one of the most important lessons I've learned is that God's will is not just something great that we aspire to do for Him, but rather it is taking whatever job God places in our hands, whether large or small, and doing it for His glory.

Caregiving is a job never aspired to and rarely trained for—one of those unexpected jobs placed in our hands by God to carry out for His glory.

2 ✳ The Mystery Woman

It's a curious trait we humans have—the desire to
be known and recognized by others.

One morning Art called out from his bedroom, "Does anyone here know me?"

We know Art, but he doesn't know us.

One of Art's frequent pastimes is saying the names of his seven children and counting them off on his fingers. He remembers them all, their full names, and repeats them over and over in birth order. But in his mind they're still children, not the gray-haired men and grown women they are today.

My husband is one of those gray-haired men. His name is Tim, but Art usually calls him Lee—who was Art's older brother and would be approaching 100 years old if he were still living. Losing his identity as a son has not been easy for Tim. Fortunately, he still rates as a family member. As for me, there is no slot for a daughter-in-law in Art's current memory bank. I am the "mystery woman" in his life.

During breakfast one morning, Art came out of his silent reverie and said, "Oh, excuse me. I haven't introduced you two."

Motioning toward Tim, he said, "This is my brother Lee."

With a nod in my direction, he said, "Lee, this is—this is—"

He hesitated and looked at me thoughtfully for a moment. Then a smile of recognition spread across his face. "This is Coffee," he said.

One day I left Art in the car for just a few seconds as I ran to do an errand. When I got back, he looked at me and said, "Oh, I'm glad it's you. There was another lady, and she was *whooee!*"

Curious, I scanned the parking lot for an unusual outfit or extreme hairdo. There was no one in sight. It suddenly dawned on me that I was the *whooee* lady!

Art finds my identity particularly perplexing when he and I are home alone. One day he came into the kitchen and quizzed me.

"Are you Leah Belle?" he asked, thinking perhaps that I was his deceased wife.

When he found out I wasn't, he went through the names of all his sons and then tried the daughters. "Are you from the Janet and Jill section?" (*section* being another all-purpose noun he uses frequently when a more specific term slips his mind.)

"No, I'm not from those sections," I replied.

"Well, whom do you represent?" he asked, thoroughly mystified.

"I'm Tim Carey's wife," I answered.

"Tim Carey?" he repeated. "Who was his father?"

"You're Tim Carey's father," I said.

"Well, that was a long time ago," he said dismissingly, as though it had nothing to do with our current conversation.

At Christmas time, all our children were home for the holidays. We were a large group around the dining room table, enjoying a leisurely breakfast one morning. When I went into the kitchen to get the coffee pot, Art told the family that the waitress was not doing a very good job keeping the cups filled.

"She must be new," he said, cutting me a little slack.

A few days later, I was doing some handwork in the living room while Art played the piano. Art spotted our daughter in the hall and called out to her, "Dear, do we have a room for this lady? She needs a place to spend the night."

"I'll check," she said.

In a few seconds she came back and reported, "Yes, we have one over there."

14

"Oh, thank you, dear," Art said, content that there was a place for the homeless waif sitting on the couch.

When I returned from shopping one morning, Art met me at the door. "Dear, out of all those people standing in line, you are the first to make it in," he congratulated.

I glanced over my shoulder. *People? In line?* I saw no one, but then it came to me—*the hedge people! Now I was one of the hedge people.*

The hedge encloses our yard and has a lockable gate—a perfect situation for taking care of Art, allowing him the freedom to roam outdoors without the danger of wandering off. But one morning I glanced out the window and saw that the gate was standing open and Art was heading out.

Oh, no! I forgot to lock it when Tim left for work. What to do now?

Taking advantage of my mysterious identity, I ran to the gate and said, "Oh, Pastor Carey, how nice of you to drop by. Do you have time for a dish of ice cream?"

Perplexed, he looked up and down the road, as though he were trying to decide—*was I coming or going?* In the end, his pastor's heart won out.

"Of course, dear," he said, as he took my arm and we headed toward the house.

Being a mystery woman does have its benefits.

Caregiver's Prayer

Dear God, protect my heart from feelings of rejection and hurt when I'm not recognized or remembered. Help me be content as an anonymous blessing to my loved one today.

3 ✳ A Cloth of All Trades

Art is from the handkerchief generation. Tucking one into his pocket is an essential step in his morning routine. He has a habit of spreading his handkerchief out to dry after using it—on the couch or over the piano—and forgetting where he put it. Getting a new one fills him with no end of wonderment over how white and fresh it looks.

I had never realized what a versatile item a handkerchief is until Art came to live with us.

Folding, unfolding, and refolding his handkerchief provides daily entertainment. For Art, the folding process is an exacting science. Once I found him sitting at the piano. He had his handkerchief stretched out over the keys and methodically went through the procedure of folding it, explaining the steps as he went.

"Yours are smaller, but you can do it the same way," Art said as he looked up at the miniature bears decorating the top of the piano.

One afternoon Art spent a good while in the bathroom. I finally went to check on him. When I opened the door, the smell told me that he had finally been successful in overcoming constipation. He was sitting there, folding and unfolding something white.

At first I thought it was toilet paper and almost shut the door. But before I did, I asked, "Do you have enough toilet paper, Art?"

"I only have this," he said forlornly. "It's tremendously nice. I think I brought it from home."

Glancing again—one doesn't just stare at an old fellow sitting on the toilet—I saw that he was holding his white handkerchief, not toilet paper.

"Oh, you can put that away, Art—here's some toilet paper," I said, offering him a new roll.

Relieved, he tucked his handkerchief in his shirt pocket and said, "Oh, thank you, dear."

Tim and I live in Guatemala. When Art came to live with us, he became an international traveler. We were going through airport security one morning when an official asked to see our identification. Tim got out his and Art's passports, and I pulled out mine. Art must have taken a cue that he needed to show something. He fumbled around in his pockets until—aha! He found his handkerchief. He carefully laid it on the counter for the official to examine.

"Dad, he doesn't want to see that," Tim said.

"I don't know why not—it's a dandy!" Art said.

There are days when Art's responsibilities weigh on his mind. One afternoon he urgently needed to leave. He had to pick up his wife, Leah Belle. He thought that perhaps he had left her in the barn. He also had a wedding to perform and was pretty sure that his cows needed milking.

No amount of reasoning or attempts to change his focus could settle him down. His dutiful heart kept him searching for a way out—an exit from reality to the imagined responsibilities outside the hedge. Back and forth he tromped from the house to the gate. He walked the whole perimeter of the yard, looking for an escape route. He shook the gate. Finally, in desperation, he mustered his final resource—his handkerchief! Waving it over the top of the gate like a white flag of surrender, he yelled, "Help! Help!"

Caregiver's Prayer

Dear God, sometimes I'm looking for an escape route, too, from the reality of caregiving to imagined peace and pleasure beyond these responsibilities. Help me keep perspective by taking consistent breaks, even though my loved one might object. Give me eyes to see the pleasures that are within reach. And may your peace rule in my heart every step of the way.

Just Between Caregivers:
The Need to Escape

There had been nothing difficult about the day. It had been an easy day of caregiving—no attempts to run away, no frantic searches, just the usual repetitive questions and lack of contact with reality. Nothing was different; nothing was hard. But by the time we sat down to dinner, I felt as if I were going to scream. When I told Tim, he was surprised.

"You're acting nice," he said.

"I might be nice on the outside, but I'm screaming on the inside."

That evening Tim sent me to my friend's house to watch a video. We sat in her quiet living room and did handwork as we watched an old movie. When we talked, it was about real things. She didn't repeat herself once. The three hours at her house were therapeutic.

Caregivers need periodic breaks in order to maintain perspective. Some caregivers feel guilty about being away from their loved one, especially if the patient objects, becomes more confused, or gets upset. An emotional decision to give in to irrational reactions will not in the end be in the best interest of the patient. Caregiving is a marathon, not a sprint. Breaks are essential so the caregiver won't wear out before the race is over.

Start planning today to take periodic breaks. Where can you go to be refreshed? Who will take care of the patient? Write out your ideas, and carry through on them.

_____

_____

_____

_____

_____

_____

_____

_____

4 ✳ The Mysterious Duo

I put on my sunglasses, propped a pair on Art's nose, and started the engine. With his long, ancient face, prominent nose, and dark lenses hiding his eyes, he looked every bit a Mafia capo—shrouding our errand day with a bit of mystery.

That day the mysterious duo was running Parties Unlimited. Holly, our youngest child, was a senior in high school, president of her class. The president needed our help.

Our first errand was the delivery of a flower arrangement and cinnamon rolls to the calculus class for a surprise party in honor of a beloved teacher. Then we rushed home to prepare for the next event—a nacho lunch in celebration of a classmate's birthday.

Leaving Art in the living room with a banana and milk for his morning snack, I flew into the kitchen to prepare food for the South of the Border party.

Art found me.

"This is all I have for lunch," he said, sadly holding up his banana.

"It's just a snack to tide you over. We'll have lunch later."

He walked out but returned numerous times, still holding his banana and forlornly repeating his assessment of the situation—his lunch was very meager fare. A man of his stature working for Parties Unlimited should be treated better than that, so Art had a full-fledged lunch before making the noon delivery.

After dropping off the Mexican cuisine, we had one more assignment—pick up a decorated cake for the honor society induction.

I parked directly in front of the bakery and opened the back hatch of the car—Parties Unlimited was ready for the cake.

As I waited for the baker to ring up the bill, I glanced out the window. *Good. Art is still in the car. If this doesn't take too long, we'll be okay.*

"Do you have someone to help you?" the baker asked as I was writing the check. "You don't want it sliding around in the car. It would be good to have someone hold it."

Good question. I glanced out the window again. Art, sunglasses in place, was scanning the parking lot.

"No, but I'll drive carefully," I answered.

The baker gallantly opened the door for me as I left with the large cake. I placed the box into the back of the car, wedging it with the jack and other trunk paraphernalia, and then gingerly lowered the hatch.

As I pulled out, the baker was still standing with the door half open, staring questioningly at us. Although it may have been my imagination, it seemed that he was casting a wordless accusation of misrepresentation of the truth in my direction.

With an apologetic smile and slight shrug of the shoulders, I drove away. That's just how it is—holding cakes is not in Art's job description.

* * *

The senior class president is not the only one who asks for help. Our elderly neighbor needed a ride to her doctor's appointment one day. Art and I put on our sunglasses and took her.

On the way home, traffic was in a terrible snarl—creeping along at five miles an hour and frequently halting altogether. Guatemalans are an impatient lot when it comes to slowing traffic. Creative drivers squeeze in between stalled lanes of vehicles in an attempt to get a car-length or two closer to their goal. We inched our way along—not just bumper to bumper, but also five cars abreast, where in reality only three lanes existed.

Pretty soon my copilot decided he had had enough. "You can just let me out here," Art said.

Not finding me amiable toward his idea, he tried again.

"What day is today?"

"Tuesday," I said.

"Tuesday? It was Saturday just one mile back!"

He had a point—if it were taking three days to go one mile, that would be a traffic jam to walk away from.

* * *

A few days later, Art and I, sunglasses in place, were in the car again and on our way. We had a long list of errands ahead of us, but we were equipped—drinks, snacks, and the indispensable large-print *Reader's Digest*.

Near the end of our errands, I realized that there was one contingency, however, that I had not planned for. Shifting uneasily in the driver's seat, I had to face the inevitable—I could not wait until we got home. I had to find a bathroom now.

But what would I do with Art?

Taking a man into the women's restroom is viewed with disapproval from members of the fairer sex. I was going to have to leave him on his own for a few minutes, but where would he be safe?

I considered my options as carefully as a woman in dire distress can.

McDonald's—I could buy Art a sundae, leave him happily eating at a table, and hope for the best. No. That would entail standing in line for food and then standing in line for a stall. No time for that. Besides, McDonald's is on a busy corner—much too chancy for a potential wanderer.

Our church! The secretary would watch Art. She's a kindly woman. It's a bit out of the way but worth the extra minutes.

As I pulled up to the church, a flapping banner proudly announced "Annual Rummage Sale—Public Welcome." Not only were they welcome, but they were there. The parking lot was filled to overflowing—not one space left.

Realizing that I had just squandered valuable minutes on a fruitless trip, visions of elementary school days came unbidden. There was a short period of time when the school administration decided that the bathrooms at my elementary school would be locked at the time of dismissal to prevent any loitering scholars from hiding out and later doing mischief. That policy was a big problem for me. Looking back, I'm sure my teacher would have had mercy. I was a conscientious student, not known for vandalism or pranks. But I never asked for special clemency. Many days I struggled home, hoping to make it in time. Usually I did, but the time that I didn't was utterly humiliating. *Was it going to happen again?*

Maybe not. It suddenly occurred to me that right around the corner was a quaint little restaurant surrounded by a large enclosed parking lot with lovely flowerbeds. Art loves flowers. He could admire the flora from the car. If he did get out, there would be a whole parking lot between him and the street. And even more important, I knew where the restroom was—right by the front door.

The mysterious duo roared into the restaurant's parking lot. Leaving my partner buckled in his seatbelt with his *Reader's Digest* in one hand and a snack in the other, I locked the doors and sprinted for the goal.

My return to the car was markedly different. Taking time to enjoy the artful landscaping of that lovely hideaway in the middle of the city, I strolled back. All was well. My elementary school nightmare had not reoccurred, and there was Art, sunglasses in place, sitting in the car, placidly munching his cookie.

Caregiver Prayer

Dear God, there are times when handling the logistics of an outing with my loved one seems as cumbersome as lugging a double mattress with me—some doors just are not made for both of us. Please give me foresight in planning and creativity in contingencies. Thank you that I can count on you to give me an extra spark of inspiration when I need it most, and on your loving watch-care to preside over every situation I face.

5 ✳ The Train from Long Beach

Family e-mails were flying back and forth the
spring before Art came to live with us. The theme
of the e-mails was—*who can take Dad this summer?*

Our reply was that it would not be convenient for us to do it. Our daughter Laurel was coming home for summer vacation and bringing two college friends with her. The three girls had chosen dietary investigations in Guatemala as their senior project. Our house would be their living quarters and base operation for the summer. Holly would be home too

No, it would not be convenient to have Art come. Our house would be full of girls and bustling with youthful activities.

Life, however, does not come in neat little packages—time for youthful activities, time for caring for the aged. What was not convenient became necessary, so the girls came, and Art came.

* * *

One afternoon the girls were in the kitchen planning meals for a feeding program when Art walked in and announced, "Girls, there's a lady upstairs who's sick. I'm going to play the piano for her."

I was proud of those girls. They did not snicker or inform him that this was a one-story house.

After he made his announcement, he went to the living room and played heartily.

A half hour later, he showed up in the kitchen again, rubbing his shoulder. "Girls, would one of you play for the lady upstairs? My arm's getting tired, but the music helps her feel better."

After finding a volunteer, Art sat down at the table, sipped some grape juice, and socialized with our visitors while out in the living room a twenty-year-old girl played for the lady upstairs in a one-story house.

* * *

Young ladies stay up later than old men. The girls were playing games in the dining room one night while Tim was helping his dad get ready for bed. As Tim was leaving the bedroom after tucking him in, Art said, "Give my regards to the ladies."

* * *

On the whole, Art was quite content that summer. He enjoyed the company of so many young ladies. But he did have one undying concern—*where is Leah Belle?* Although his wife had died two years before, she had never died in his mind.

"Have you seen Leah Belle?" Art asked one afternoon.

"She died two years ago," I replied. "She's in heaven."

"That's impossible—I spent all morning with her!" Art said, looking at me as though I were the one with dementia.

Another day, Art was searching for his car keys. "Leah Belle is alone. I need to go get her."

"Oh, she's not alone—she's with her brother and sister," I answered. It was true. They were all in heaven.

"How do you know?" Art asked. "Did they call?"

Truth be told—I hadn't received any calls from heaven that day.

One morning Holly was sitting at the breakfast table when Art came in and asked, "Dear, have you seen Leah Belle?"

"No, Grandpa," Holly said. "She died two years ago."

Art continued his search, as though being dead had nothing to do with her whereabouts there in the house.

A few minutes later, he came back. "Dear, have you seen Leah Belle?"

"She's in heaven, Grandpa," Holly repeated. "She died two years ago."

Completely ignoring her answer, he headed toward the back door. "I'll see if she's outside," he said.

Soon he was back. "Have you seen Leah Belle?" he asked, yet again.

Since the truth was not working, Holly tried a different tactic. "She's asleep, Grandpa. We need to be quiet so we won't wake her up."

Art put his hands on his hips. "You just told me she was dead!" he said, thoroughly scandalized.

One day Art searched high and low for Leah Belle, and I mean low. He even checked under the tablecloth on a small end table in the living room.

He searched all morning, frantic to find her. By afternoon, his quest had turned into an urgent need to get to Long Beach, where he thought she might be. He walked down to the gate, back to the house, and down to the gate again and again.

Finally I convinced him to sit on the couch and rest a minute. He put his head in his hands. "I have to get to Long Beach, but I can't quite seem to get there," he said dejectedly.

"Would you like me to take you in my car?" I asked.

He lifted his head and looked at me earnestly. "You'll take me to Long Beach? You're not lying?"

"I'll take you home," I promised.

As I was getting my keys to take Art for a drive, I overheard one of the girls say, "Boy, someday I hope I find a man who's so committed to me that two years after I'm dead, he's still looking for me."

* * *

One day Tim took the girls on an outing to the beach, and Art and I stayed home. That afternoon Art awoke from his nap with a pressing concern: the train from Long Beach was coming, and we needed to be ready.

"Do we have enough beds for everyone?" Art asked.

I took him on a tour of the house and showed him all the beds.

"Landees!" Art said, impressed. "Do we have enough blankets?"

"Oh, yes. We have plenty."

He followed me into the kitchen, "But do we have enough food?"

Stew for dinner was simmering in the Crock-Pot. I lifted the lid. "Will this be enough?" I asked.

He looked at it with the experienced eye of a maitre d' and then gave me the nod of approval. Yes, it would do.

For the rest of the afternoon, he paced through the house making sure that all was ready—accommodations and food—for the guests who would soon be arriving on the train from Long Beach.

When Tim and the girls returned home, Art met them at the door. Like a hotel concierge, he graciously welcomed the weary travelers. The train from Long Beach had arrived!

* * *

That summer was quite a jumble of youthful activities and geriatric concerns. In the end, I think it was that unique blend that made the time so special for all of us.

Caregiver Prayer

Dear God, your plan of having generations live together on the earth is good. Thank you that the liveliness of youth can bless and encourage the aged—and that young people can learn from the elderly, even those with dementia. In Jesus' name I pray. Amen.

6 ＊ Nighttime Woes

To be able to go to bed at night, drift into the unconscious state of sleep, dream of adventures far and wide, and awaken eight hours later, refreshed and ready for a new day—that was a luxury we took for granted until Art came to live with us.

We put a nightlight in Art's bedroom and one in the bathroom, guiding stars to lead him in the night. Even with that, he gets confused.

It's not uncommon for the ceiling light in our bedroom to suddenly flash on in the middle of the night, accompanied by Art's voice saying, "Is this my place?"

One night I heard the shuffling of feet, the closing of the bathroom door, and then the flush of the toilet. The door opened and all was quiet for a few moments. There was no sound of his steps returning to his bedroom—nothing. Then I heard Art's voice. "Eenie, meenie, minie, moe. Which way do I go?"

It is not just the getting back and forth to the bathroom that awakens us, but sometimes Art has occupations or worries that concern him in the night.

"Is that Art?" I asked Tim at 3 A.M.

"Yes," Tim replied, "he's been singing and talking for about two hours now."

A few nights later, I heard a voice. It was Art again. This time he was spelling, and that was more distracting than the singing and talking. I found myself straining from my bed to decipher what the letters spelled.

One night Art was calling out, "Hello! Hello! Are you there?"

I went to check on him. He was just feeling lonely and wanted to talk. When his conversation turned to two horses that he thought he may have left in a field, I heard sniggering coming from our daughters' room. Holly and Laurel obviously had been awakened too.

Somehow it's easier to face challenges in the night as a team. The combined brainpower comes up with more creative solutions. The girls cranked up their CD player with some soft instrumental hymns, and Art happily hummed for about an hour and then went back to sleep.

A few nights later, I heard Art and our daughter talking in the wee hours of the morning. I hopped out of bed to see what was up. He was frantic. Someone was taking people away. Where was Leah Belle? Where was his little girl? For that matter, where were all the things that used to be in his room? What if they came for him next?

"Everything's okay, Grandpa," Holly said. "Go back to bed. See you in the morning."

"I hope I'll be here in the morning," Art said. "You never can tell about the Greeks."

We finally convinced him to get back in bed. As we were walking out of the room, Art said, "If you hear a yelp, come with your base—your base—"

"Baseball bat?" Holly asked.

"Yes, baseball bat," Art said, relieved that she had guessed the right word.

* * *

It was 2 A.M. I heard voices. It was Art and Tim.

"I'm going to die. There's no food. I'm going to die," Art said.

"Stop saying that—you're not going to die," Tim said. "You have had plenty to eat."

Then it was quiet, and Tim came back to bed. "I found one of his Christmas chocolates on his nightstand, unwrapped it, and stuck it in his mouth," Tim said wearily.

All was quiet for about as long as it takes to eat a Hershey's Kiss. Then we heard a melancholy voice singing, "The food is gone. There's no more. The food is gone."

* * *

One of the Proverbs of Solomon says that a righteous man cares for the needs of his animal. Art is a righteous man.

The dog next door is a pit bull that has a propensity for barking, especially at night. The wire fence and our cypress hedge do little to mute the noise. Tim and I have become accustomed to ignoring the racket, but any barking dog is a concern to Art.

One night when the pit bull was barking furiously, we heard the front door open and a tremulous voice call, "Sheppy! Sheppy! Come in, Sheppy."

Tim got up and helped Art back to bed.

Twenty minutes later, we heard the shuffling of feet, the opening of the door, and the same voice, calling, "Pudge! Pudge! Come in, Pudge." Art's mind was ambling over memories of dogs long gone as he wandered through the house, intent on being a righteous man.

A few months later, Tim heard the front door open in the middle of the night and found Art in his pajamas, wanting to take care of the dog.

"Dad, it's the neighbor's dog that's barking—it's not our dog," Tim said as he escorted Art back to bed.

The barking continued, and it was not long until we heard Art opening the front door again.

"Dad, you need to get back to bed," Tim said.

"The dog is hungry. We need to feed him," Art replied.

"Dad, it's the neighbor's dog that's barking. Our dog died a long time ago."

"Well, this one will, too, if we don't feed it," Art said.

* * *

One day the pit bull broke through the chain link fence into our yard. In an attempt to prevent it from happening again, our neighbors tried an unusual tactic. They lined the fence with tin roofing. The pit bull developed the obnoxious habit of leaping against the fence. The noise was deafening.

Before dawn one morning, the dog was making a terrible ruckus, jumping against the fence and barking wildly. We heard Art call out, and Tim went to settle him down.

He sat down on the edge of Art's bed and said, "Don't worry about the dog. He's okay. He probably sees an animal—a possum or something—and is trying to get at it."

"What are we going to do with them?" Art said.

"With whom?" Tim asked.

"Oh, I don't know—cats, maybe," Art replied.

Tim explained again that the dog next door was trying to get some animal and was crashing into the fence.

"Probably the cat," Art said.

Trying to change the subject in hopes of being able to get back to bed sometime soon, Tim told Art that his second son was having a birthday that very day. "He's sixty-five years old today," Tim said, thinking that should be impressive enough to draw Art's attention to a new topic.

"Well, let's give him the cat!" Art said.

It's difficult to know how to handle our nighttime woes when we're only half awake and dead tired.

Give him the cat. Now that's a creative solution.

Caregiver's Prayer

Dear God, I desperately need your help. It's so easy to become frustrated and angry when my loved one is up and down in the night. I get so tired and say things that I really regret. In the midnight hours, give wisdom to my foggy brain and patience to my weary heart. And, Lord, please help us to get a good night's rest tonight.

Just Between Caregivers
Safety for Midnight Wanderers

1. Assure that the patient cannot leave the house. Some options for securing outside access doors include changing the locks to a type that requires a key for exit and entry or installing a sliding bolt at floor level.
2. Use infant gates to close off stairs or parts of the house that are off limits to your loved one.
3. Put nightlights in the bathroom, bedroom, and hall.
4. Remove floor clutter and small area rugs that could cause stumbling in the dark.

7 ✳ The Novel

I love reading. Hand me a novel, and I'm off on a
new adventure to places I've never been.

Living with Art is like opening a new book every day or sometimes several books in a day. As with any novel, it takes a while to identify characters, setting, and plot.

Art was lying down for a nap when Holly heard him call out. She went to see what he wanted.

"I'm feeling great," Art said to her. "There's nothing wrong with me. Can I go now? That other guy over there is pretty bad, but I'm fine."

Setting: A hospital room

Characters: Holly, a nurse

       Art, a patient

       An anonymous male patient

Plot: Art wants to be released from the hospital.

The whereabouts of the anonymous male patient were quite a mystery. There's only one bed in Art's room.

* * *

One evening we were returning from Holly's afternoon basketball game. Art and Tim were in the front seat, and Holly and I were in the back.

"Lee, we need to drop them off at the dorm," Art said. "It's getting late, and the cafeteria is going to close."

Characters: Art and Tim, college boys

       Holly and I, college girls

Plot: Art and Tim need to get to the cafeteria, without

       girls, before it closes.

That storyline made middle-aged caregivers feel young. It also alerted us that Art was getting hungry.

Tim pulled into the Burger King parking lot, and we college kids piled out. Tim and I stepped up to the counter, and Holly and Art stood behind us.

While we were ordering, Art searched all his pockets. Then he whispered to Holly, "Dear, I don't have any money."

Holly patted all of her pockets and said, "I don't have any either. Let's stick together."

She locked arms with Art and led him to a table where those two conspirators hid out and waited for their more affluent friends to bring them food.

❊ ❊ ❊

Art was in a dither.

"I can't find that outfit for my neck," he said. Then he rubbed his already shaven face. "Oh, no. I better shave. That young couple will be here soon."

He picked up an old copy of *Decision* magazine and flipped anxiously through it. "I've got to find something good," he said. "You can't say just anything on their special day."

Aha! Wedding bells were ringing in his mind.

Character: Art, a pastor.

Setting: The parsonage.

Plot: A young couple is coming to be married.

❊ ❊ ❊

One morning Art found me in the kitchen. "Would you come see if it's working better?" he said.

He led me to the piano and asked me to sit down on the bench and play something.

As a child, I took six years of piano lessons. Unfortunately, I was neither a gifted nor dedicated student. Now as an adult, I play only one song—a very simplified and extremely slow version of "O Holy Night."

Art waited expectantly while I struggled through it.

"I think it needs a little more work," he said pensively at the end of my torturous journey through the carol.

Thankfully, at that moment it was Art who needed to do more work, not the novice pianist. He sat down and slowly played a number of arpeggios, listening carefully. Then he played a few chords, tisking and clucking about the quality of the sound.

I think I have it, I thought.

Characters: Art, a piano repairman

              Me, owner of the piano

Plot: Art is tuning my piano.

It seemed like a harmless storyline since he was not trying to open the piano, nor did he have any tools.

But a few minutes later, he came in and said, "Dear, I think I'm finished. I've put black spots on all the keys, and they're working fine now."

Black spots on the keys? Oh, no!

Horrified, I ran to the living room and was tremendously relieved to find no visible black spots on white keys. His failing eyesight and confused mind must have jumbled up white and black keys. All was well, but maybe it was time for him to read a story rather than act one out.

I sat him down with a book, but it wasn't long until Art came into the kitchen.

"Good-bye," he said.

"Where are you going?" I asked.

"To join my group," he responded.

After some talking, I deciphered that we had moved on to a new novel.

Character: Art, a soldier.

Plot: Art has become separated from his regiment and
              needs to rejoin them.

* * *

One night as we were starting dinner, Art turned to Tim and asked, "Do I go in now?"

Tim, thinking that Art, with his failing vocabulary, was asking whether he should start eating, said, "Yes—go ahead."

Art got up and started to walk away.

"Dad, where are you going?"

"In. You said I was supposed to go in."

"No, no. Sit down. I thought you were asking if you were supposed to eat now."

"Well, will he come out?" asked Art.

"No, he won't come out," Tim said with certainty, yet wondering who in the world "he" was.

"Well, will his inside come out?" Art replied.

"No," Tim said, "Please, just eat."

Art sat there eating and then mumbled, "I wonder when the doc will see me."

Suddenly we had it figured out.

Characters: Art, a patient waiting to see the doctor.

Tim, accompanying family member.

Setting: The doctor's waiting room.

What a waiting room! An eat-a-hot-meal-while-you-wait waiting room.

"When will the doc eat?" Art asked.

"Oh, when he has time," Tim replied.

It's easier to answer when you know the characters and setting.

"Is he having trouble with the guy in there?" Art said.

"Maybe."

Dinner conversation was a cyclic repetition of questions regarding the doctor, his current patient, and the possibility of Art ever getting his turn. When Art's plate was empty, he got up and headed off toward the guestroom.

Finding it dark, he came back, discouraged. "How am I going to find the doc?" he said.

"Are you sick?" I asked, wondering if perhaps the reason for this storyline was because he wasn't feeling well.

"Did you say 'sick' or 'thick'?" Art replied.

"'Sick.' S—I—C—K," I spelled.

"Oh, thick. Yes, I'm thick," he said, leaving the room, a disappointed patient.

With that, the novel of *The Waiting Room* ended. It remains to be seen what our next novel will be.

Caregiver's Prayer

Dear God, you are the author of life. As I face the uncertainty and frustrations of each day, keep my focus on you and the role you have for me—not a harried, hopeless individual but a person of faith who finds strength, joy, and peace in you.

Just Between Caregivers
Knowledge of the Past May Unlock Mysteries of Today

Write down what you know of your patient's personal history, such as jobs, hobbies, and travels. These may be helpful clues for understanding your patient's mental wanderings.

_____

_____

_____

_____

_____

_____

8 ✳ The Radio Program

Art is a pianist. As a child, he spent hours pumping the pedals of his family's player piano, watching the keys, and then imitating what he saw. It was an unusual method for learning to play, but it worked for Art. To this day, his style is like that of a player piano, with fancy runs and rich chords.

Playing the piano provides Art with hours of entertainment and fills our home with joyous, albeit repetitious music.

One morning the piano music stopped, and I heard the bench scrape on the tile floor—my cue to check on Art.

I peeked into the living room. Art was alone in the room, standing at attention beside the piano.

"I'm Reverend Carey," he said as enthusiastically as a ninety-five year old man can. "I'm pastor of the church here. We have Sunday School classes for all ages. Come and bring the whole family." Then he sat down at the piano and played with gusto, only to stop, stand again, and give another rambling account about the activities at his church.

This was a perplexing twist to his usual piano playing. Obviously, Reverend Carey was the character, and the setting was his church. The plot, however, was a mystery.

A few days later, it happened again. But that time, instead of standing, Art remained seated on the piano bench. He played, then talked about his church, then played again. When he talked, he lifted his head toward the cone-shaped lamp on top of the piano, as though he were talking into it. He ended his narration this time with "Well, folks, I hope you'll tune in again tomorrow."

Tune in? Tune in! That's it!

Character: Reverend Carey

Plot: Reverend Carey hosts a radio program.

Art must have quite a contract with the radio station, because he's on the air frequently.

During one afternoon broadcast I heard him say, "We have an exciting youth rally going on here today. Come on down to the church and join us."

I looked around at the youth present—ninety-five-year-old Art and middle-aged me. Some youth rally!

* * *

One night Art was restless. He was in and out of bed numerous times, wearing us to a frazzle. Finally Tim gave him some bread and milk, hoping that a little nourishment would settle him down.

The snack only served as inspiration for a 1 A.M. radio broadcast. Art took the bread and thought he was supposed to read something off it to his audience. The glass of milk became his microphone. He lifted it to his mouth at a daring angle and began his program. But that was as far as he got. Tim hustled him back to bed before he could spill his milk or bless his audience with midnight medleys on the piano.

* * *

One morning Art was having a very long and repetitious program. He talked and talked to his radio audience, encouraging them to come to his church. He even invited his listeners to call into the program. His broadcast went on for more than an hour.

I didn't mind. I was in the middle of a painting project and was relieved that he was occupied and enjoying himself.

While the radio preacher droned on and on, I painted the dining room and then went to the utility room to wash out my roller. When I came back, Art was standing by the piano beaming.

"I had a call-in!" he announced joyfully.

"You did?" I said incredulously.

"Yes! It was the daughter of a friend of mine. I didn't know her, but it was so nice of her to call in."

I had come to accept Art's radio programs as part and parcel of his dementia. But call-ins? His flights of fantasy were taking him too far!

In the afternoon, the phone rang. It was my friend.

"Oh, I'm so glad it's you!" she said. "When I called this morning, Art answered on the first ring."

She had told Art that she was a friend of his daughter-in-law. That's pretty close to what Art heard—a daughter of his friend.

She said that Art had been very cordial but, of course, didn't know anyone by my name. We laughed about how she should have asked for Mystery Woman or Coffee, and finally moved on to the topic that she had originally called to discuss.

When I hung up, I checked on Art, who was lying down for his afternoon nap. He was sound asleep.

I can't believe it, I thought. *You really* did *have a call-in.*

Caregiver Prayer

Dear God, it's me—calling in! Thank you that you offer wise counsel when I don't know what to do, comfort when I'm sad, and peace when I'm frustrated. In this job of caregiving, I'm never alone. You're my ever-present help. Thank you for your open invitation to call on you anytime, night or day. In Jesus' name I pray. Amen.

9 ✳ My Neighbor

My masterpiece—a baby quilt with an intricate appliqué design—was nearing completion. I was closing in on the finish line and just in time. The baby shower was that night. Hunched over the sewing machine, I imagined the oohs and ahhs I would hear from the ladies when my exquisite gift was opened.

Art's voice jerked me back to reality. "Who will milk the cows?" he asked.

Reality? What do the agricultural worries of a ninety-five-year-old city dweller have to do with reality?

It is the reality of caregiving.

Hoping to quickly calm his concerns and get back to work, I gave an answer that would have rung with veracity during the farm days of his youth.

"Your brothers will take care of everything," I said,

"But do they know that I'm not on the farm?" he asked.

"Everyone in the family knows you're not on the farm," I said, thankful for a question that I could answer in the here-and-now with all honesty.

"The chickens can't get out of the chicken coop."

"Everything is fine," I said. "Don't worry."

"No, don't worry about it—just let them die," he said disgustedly as he tromped out of the guestroom.

He was upset, just as a good farmer would be if he thought his animals were not being cared for.

A few minutes later I heard an odd noise from the dining room. I went to check, and there was Art, all tangled up in the draperies, trying to find a way to the farm.

I guided him to the front door and opened it. The gate was locked. He could not escape. Maybe roaming outside would relieve his agrarian concerns.

He went out the front door and soon came in the back door, mumbling about the farm. He went out again and returned with some greenery stuck on his sweater.

I looked at the sprig of cypress in amazement. *Where has he been? The hedge! He must have been trying to get out through the hedge.* No doubt about it—he was desperate to get to the farm.

He'll be okay—he can't get out, I assured myself as I returned to the sewing machine. But my heart was not at peace. My Bible study of the night before was running through my mind.

"How would you define 'neighbor'?" the leader had asked as she guided us through a discussion of the Good Samaritan. After some debate, we had come up with a definition: My neighbor— any human being who needs my help.

Any human being who needs my help, I mused. *Today that would be Art.* Although his agricultural duties were imaginary, his agitation and frustration were very real. He needed help.

I unplugged the iron, turned off the sewing machine light, and shut the door, not only on the guestroom, but also on the possibility of giving the quilt as a gift that night.

I found my neighbor outside, searching for a breach in the hedge.

"Let's go," I said, holding open the door of the car.

He came quickly. Obviously, "go" in his mind implied "to the farm."

The bumpy road out of our neighborhood was like driving through the autumn stubble of an Ohio cornfield, but the farm of Art's youth was far, far away, both in miles and decades. An alternative destination would have to do.

I drove to the shopping center, where we meandered through various stores. In one, I bought a fluffy sleeper—a substitute present for the baby shower.

The coffee shop was running a special on coffee and donuts. When the waitress brought our order, she patted Art on the shoulder. "How are you doing?" she asked.

"Oh, we're having a wonderful day," said my neighbor, whose agricultural worries had drifted away.

* * *

Maria, who is a mere four foot, ten inches tall, works at our house a few days a week, allowing me periodic breaks from caregiving. The little dynamo has a loving, patient heart, and in spite of her limited English, she finds ways to communicate with Art.

When she arrived for work the day after the shower, I told her about my Bible study on the parable of the Good Samaritan and the adventures of the day before with my neighbor.

"Art is going to be your neighbor today," I said. "I'm going to shut myself in the guestroom and work on my project. Just pretend that I'm not here unless there's an emergency."

I entered the guestroom with a sack lunch and a thermos of coffee—armed to stay the whole day—and shut the door.

While Maria took care of Art, I finished the quilt, not emerging from my cloister until late afternoon when it was time for her to go home.

My day in seclusion had been so peaceful that I assumed Maria's had been too. But on the dining room table I found a three-by-five card with the words "They are trees." The handwriting was Maria's. Curious, I asked her about it.

"Oh, Art wouldn't sit down to eat," she said. "He wanted the hedge people to join us for lunch. I tried to talk to him, but he couldn't understand me. So I wrote the note. It worked. He read it, laughed, sat down, and ate."

Maria is a creative neighbor.

*   *   *

A neighborhood is a reciprocal community.

The phone rang early one morning.

"Bring Art over today and take a break," the Good Samaritan said.

I had an extra day in my life—a free day to do whatever I wanted. It was exhilarating.

I called my hairdresser and made an appointment.

While she was cutting my hair, she asked about Art. I told her about the friend who was caring for him, giving me an unexpected day of freedom.

As I was leaving, she handed me a gift card from her salon for a free pedicure. "Give this to your friend, a thank-you from me for taking care of Art," she said.

Small ripples of kindness I had shown to my neighbor seemed insignificant as waves of thoughtfulness from others in the neighborhood washed over me.

Caregiver's Prayer

Dear God, thank you for the Good Samaritans who have reached out to me to lighten my load and brighten my days. Protect my heart from being judgmental or bitter toward those who are too busy or blind to see my need. Give me humility and grace to accept the love and help offered by those who do. Help me live fully in the neighborhood you've placed me in—reaching out as a good neighbor and gratefully receiving the neighborliness of others.

10 ✳ The "Don'tist"

The international phone line crackled. "He needs
a physical and a tuberculin tine test." It was Tim's
brother in California, who had offered to take care
of Art while we visited my parents. He was making arrangements for Art to attend the Salvation
Army adult daycare center during work hours.
Before Art could be accepted into the program,
there were requirements to be met.

The form for the physical arrived in the mail, and I made an appointment with our family physician.

Guatemalans have an appreciation for the elderly that approaches reverence. When we entered the examining room, Dr. Ramirez gallantly rose from his chair and shook Art's hand.

"It's an honor to meet you, Mr. Carey," he said in impeccable English that he had perfected in his days of internship in the United States.

I handed him the form that asked for an assessment of Art's mental as well as physical status. After a quick perusal of the document, the doctor looked at Art and said, "Well, Mr. Carey, can you tell me what year this is?"

Art shifted in his chair and gave me a worried glance, but I smiled encouragingly.

"1927," he said, giving it his best shot.

Further questioning revealed that Harry Truman currently sat in the Oval Office.

As the interview continued, Art warmed to the task. He was enjoying talking to this genial man who was so interested in him. He even started offering random information.

"My name is Art, but sometimes they call me other things," he said, and then proceeded to list both the first and middle names of his five sons.

Our doctor did not have the tuberculin tine test on hand, so he called another doctor who was sure to have a supply.

"Go to office 306—they'll be expecting you," he said. He shook Art's hand and bid us goodbye.

"I hate to leave," Art replied. "I'm having such a good time."

We rode the elevator to the third floor and found suite 306. I opened the door and started to walk in but quickly stepped back to recheck the number. It was no mistake. This was 306.

The waiting room walls were decorated with giraffes, elephants, and monkeys cavorting in a jungle setting. A television set suspended from the wall played an episode of SpongeBob Squarepants as a band of preschoolers scrimmaged over some red-and-blue blocks on the floor. A distraught mother paced back and forth with her wailing baby.

I told the receptionist Art's name, and she said, "Oh, yes—your doctor just called. Our inoculation nurse will be with you in a minute."

I steered Art toward the only seating that was left—a red vinyl couch that must have been special-ordered by a dwarf.

Soon a nurse stepped out and called, "Art Carey."

Art's shuffle to the inoculation room was viewed with unabashed astonishment by the adults in the room. It was not long until Art himself was astounded. The nurse, accustomed to dealing with wiggly children, was lightning fast.

"What did I do to deserve that?" asked Art who at that moment could have gained a spot in the Guinness World Records as the oldest pediatric patient in the world.

Art soon forgot the jab. But on the way home, he incredibly remembered his visit with our friendly family doctor and had some concerns over my forgetfulness.

"Dear," he said, "I think you forgot to tell him that I'm a reverend."

* * *

There was another medical visit that jogged Art's mind into an exceptionally long stretch of mental acuity.

"Art, please brush your teeth. You have a dentist appointment this afternoon."

"Dentist!" Art replied with vigor. "I don't need a dentist."

He *did* need a dentist. One tooth had broken, and a part of it had slipped sideways, gouging the gum and causing considerable pain.

Art, like most of us, is afraid of dentists, and fear is not easily forgotten.

"If the dentist wants my teeth clean, he can clean them himself," Art said, still refusing to brush his teeth.

Better to drop the matter, I thought. *He'll forget, and I'll just load him in the car. We'll go to the dentist without brushing.*

"Why don't you play the piano?" I suggested.

As the music started, I went back to the salad I was making for supper.

It wasn't long until I heard the scraping of the piano bench on the floor, and Art came to the kitchen in search of me.

"Who wants me to go to the dentist anyway?" Art asked, still remembering.

"Your son, Tim," I replied.

"Well, if he wants me to go, why doesn't he come and take me?"

"We are going to meet him at his office, and he'll take you from there," I said, thankful that we had a plan that included Tim.

I sat Art down at the kitchen table with a book to read, but he could not forget the upcoming dentist appointment.

"My teeth are perfectly fine. They never give me any trouble. I don't want any dentist grinding away on perfectly good teeth."

When it was time to go, I loaded Art in the car. He did not mention the dentist.

Good—he's finally forgotten, I thought.

When he started whistling in the car, I was certain that his dental concerns had evaporated into the blur of dementia. But after a few rounds of medleys, he looked at me forlornly. "I've got to do it now, because I won't be able to after the dentist."

We wove in and out of traffic. Art stopped whistling and quietly watched the hubbub around him, but he didn't forget the dentist or the fact that he had not brushed his teeth.

"I didn't brush my teeth. Now that dentist will charge me fifty cents to clean them," he complained.

When we came to a section of road riddled by potholes, Art decided that he might not have any teeth left for the dentist to clean after all, but he was not resigned to his fate.

He had one final objection. "A dentist should be called a 'don'tist,' because I don't want to go."

Having released his frustration as forcefully as his pious nature would allow, he lapsed into forgetfulness.

At the dentist's office, he happily climbed into the dental chair, mentioning that he did indeed need a haircut. Even when his teeth became the center of attention rather than his hair, he sat there like a model citizen and endured the procedure without complaint. Oh, the bliss of dementia!

Caregiver Prayer

Dear God, keep my eyes and ears alert to clues that my loved one needs medical attention, since his expressing those needs is no longer possible. Lead us to perceptive medical personnel who can read between the lines and diagnose adequately. Help me carry out my role as patient advocate with a balanced blend of graciousness and firmness.

Just Between Caregivers
A Special Bag for Medical Appointments

When our children were young, I had a picnic basket that I kept packed for doctor appointments. In it I had cups, packaged snacks, and special little toys like a kaleidoscope, a View-Master with disks of pictures to insert, felt shapes and a little flannel board, and a miniature blackboard and colored chalk. The pediatrician's receptionist commented one afternoon on how well-behaved my children were. They were calm and content because their needs were being met—thanks to the basket.

Similarly, having a special bag packed and ready for medical appointments or emergency room visits can make the experience much more pleasant for an Alzheimer's patient and the caregiver.

The bag should include—

1. **A sweater**. Feeling cold in an air-conditioned office makes the dementia patient eager to leave.

2. **A snack** that the patient likes and can easily eat; low blood sugar creates anxiety.

3. **A plastic cup**. Paper cones at water fountains and water bottles are sometimes difficult for the dementia patient to manage.

4. **Entertainment**. A large-print *Reader's Digest* was adequate entertainment for Art. My friend packed colorful kerchiefs, because her mother liked to fold and unfold things.

5. **An envelope-type folder** or a folder with pockets to hold lab requests and prescriptions that the doctor might give. The folder should always have—

   a. **A current list of the patient's medications**. Be sure to include dosage and frequency.

   b. **The patient's Medicare and insurance cards**.

11 ✳ Locked In, Locked Out

"Dear, do you have a map?" Art asked one day.

"Why?" I asked.

He looked wistful. "If I had a map, I could find my way home."

Home is sometimes in California, sometimes in Ohio, but always somewhere beyond the hedge. Art is searching for a place where his heart will say, *Ah, I'm home.* Without memory, it's an insatiable quest. That's why we lock the gate.

The gate was locked when I returned home from my Friday morning Bible study. I pushed the button to announce my arrival.

I waited and waited. No one answered the intercom; no one came.

You might wonder why I didn't pull out a key and let myself in. Our locked gate is more complicated than that.

Seismic conditions in our part of the world have caused the doorposts of the gate to shift, and the metal doors no longer meet in the middle. Due to the gap, a conventional deadbolt lock—one that a key can open and shut from both sides—is not an option. We have resorted to a more primitive solution—a metal bar that slides between the two doors and is secured with padlocks. The only way to lock or unlock the gate is from the inside.

Maria had secured the padlocks when I left that morning. *Where was she now?*

I checked my watch. It was almost noon. The doorbell is connected to a phone-like intercom in the kitchen. She should be in the kitchen making lunch for Art. *Why wasn't she answering?*

I pushed the button again.

Nothing.

Having imbibed two cups of coffee at the Bible study, I was beginning to feel the effects of that natural diuretic. I punched the button again and held it down for a full thirty seconds.

"Hello."

Oh, no! Why was Art answering the intercom?

"Art, I need to talk to Maria."

"What? I can't hear you."

"I need to talk to the lady!" I yelled in staccato-fashion into the flat box over the doorbell.

"No lady here."

"Yes, there is!" I hollered back. "Please go look for her!"

"It's lunchtime. Everybody's gone to lunch." Art might forget many things, but he knows when it's time to eat.

"Art, please go look for the lady! Art? Art!"

All was silent. Was he searching for her? Even if he was, it's one thing to head out with a mission in mind, but to carry through with that mission takes a lot of memory cells.

I pounded on the gate. Still no one came.

Something was wrong with this picture. The padlocks were for keeping Art in, not me out. But there I stood—locked out of my own yard. What was I going to do?

In fourth grade I enjoyed moderate success as a hurdler for my elementary school track team, better known as the Taft Rockets.

I stepped back and contemplated the gate. Could I scale that five-and-a-half-foot barrier?

For someone lighter and more agile, perhaps climbing over would be a possibility. But hefting my matronly body over that formidable barricade would take Herculean strength. It was utterly impossible, even for an ex-Rocketeer like me.

With a final push on the doorbell, which still proved to be futile, I got in the car and drove to a nearby school—my children's alma mater. There I used the restroom and called home. Fortunately, Maria answered the phone, and the gate was wide open when I returned.

All was well, except the episode left me with a niggling doubt about how well Maria was caring for Art in my absence. Was she attentive enough? There's something about being a caregiver that makes you feel that no one can do the job quite as well as you do.

* * *

A few months later, Tim was asked to do a guest appearance on a local television station. The morning of his debut, he dressed in his best—a dark gray suit, starched white shirt, and smartly polished shoes.

I sent the impressive personage on his way, put the padlocks on the gate, and headed for the computer. I had a deadline to meet—a finance report was due at noon. Hunched over the computer keyboard, I totally lost track of time as I wrestled with complicated formulas and frustrating totals.

A male voice pulled me from my silent reverie. "What are you doing?"

Startled, I whipped around, and there was Tim standing in the doorway of the office—his white shirt smudged with dirt, his tie askew, and his shoes scuffed.

"What happened to you?"

"That's what I was wondering about you," he said. "I've been ringing the bell and pounding the gate for the last ten minutes."

He further informed me that when he looked through the gap in the gate, he could see Art on the front step trying to get into the house.

Spurred by his fear that something was amiss and being much more athletic than his wife, he had then vaulted over the gate, suit and all.

I glanced at the clock. Over two hours had passed since I gave Art his snack. Sometime after that, he must have gone out the front door and shut it behind him—locking himself out.

How long had he been out there?

I didn't know. I had been totally oblivious.

It was a low moment in my caregiving career.

But one good thing came out of it. My egotistical thought that no one could do the job as well as I was put to rest permanently.

Caregiver Prayer

Dear God, I confess that I'm not a perfect caregiver. Forgive my times of negligence and impatience. Deliver me from the futility of wallowing in guilt when I fall short. Give me insight to learn from my mistakes and courage to continue on—a better, wiser person. In Jesus' name I pray. Amen.

Just Between Caregivers
Being Less than Perfect

My father once said, "If you're going to look back only to feel bad, don't look back. But if in looking back you can learn from your mistakes—look back, learn, and go on."

Have you had times when you felt like a failure as a caregiver? What wisdom can you gain from those situations that will help you do better in the future?

_____

_____

_____

_____

_____

_____

_____

12 ✳ A Tenacious Little Dog

"There's a dog on the hood of the car," Art stated as I fastened my seat belt.

"A dog? On the hood of the car?" I asked in disbelief.

"Yes, he's right there," he said, pointing to the windshield.

I looked and saw nothing, but all the way to the store, Art gave me a running commentary on the state of the dog.

"He's black and white. He's a little one."

"How does he stay on there? Go slow! He might fall off."

"Oh, he's running on the road now."

"No, he's back on the hood."

"Wait—no, he's running on the road again."

"Oh, no! You're going to hit him. Watch out!"

That invisible little dog was making me a nervous wreck with his antics!

I tried changing the subject, hoping that Art would forget about the dog. But that pesky mutt stayed right with us—hopping from the hood to the road and back to the hood again, imperiling his life and ours too.

Finally we arrived at the grocery store and went in. We walked up and down every aisle with Art pushing the cart and adding a few groceries when I wasn't looking. The whole time we were shopping, he did not mention a dog, not even once.

I was relieved. Finally something had loosened that canine's hold on Art's mind. But no! The minute we got into the car, the acrobatic dog was back.

How can he forget so much and yet remember a dog that doesn't exist? I wondered as Art resumed his monologue.

"He's running on the road."

"Watch out!"

"He's going to get hit. That car is coming straight at him."

"Oh, good—he's back on the hood!" he said with relief, as though having a dog jump onto the hood of a moving car was a perfectly normal thing.

"No, he's on the road. He's running."

"He's getting tired. Poor thing."

"See that blue car? They're the owners of that dog. Why don't they stop and let him in? He's been running so hard and so long."

Art kept up his banter about the dog so persistently that he had to be seeing something, but what was it?

There was a slowdown in traffic, so I decided to do some investigation. I began moving my hand in front of the windshield on the passenger's side of the car.

At one point Art exclaimed, "Oh, he's gone."

I moved my hand to another location.

"He's back."

I returned my hand to the previous location.

"He's gone again."

I removed my hand.

"There he is! He's back!" Art chuckled with relief.

Aha! I had found it. The windshield had a splotch of bird droppings—black and white—our tenacious little dog.

Caregiver's Prayer

Dear God, protect me from "What if" and "If only" thoughts that keep me from experiencing the joy of today. Give me a heart of contentment, and keep my sense of humor intact.

13 ✳ Choir Practice

"I'm going to take that bone off your plate," I said, reaching over to remove a chicken bone from Art's plate.

"There's a barn on my plate?" he asked.

"No, a bone," I said.

"Oh, ho!" He chuckled, happy that he had finally figured out what I was trying to say. "A bomb! I thought that you said 'a barn'!"

Dementia plus poor eyesight plus partial deafness equals unusual dinner conversations.

* * *

On Thursday evenings the single teachers who work at a Christian school nearby have a standing invitation to come to our house for dinner. It's a custom I started years ago when I taught at the school. Even though I'm no longer teaching, the tradition continues.

One Thursday night, three young ladies joined us for supper. They entertained us with stories from their classrooms and then started talking about an upcoming wedding.

"I'm having trouble deciding on bridesmaids' dresses," said the soon-to-be bride.

"The color?" I asked.

"No, the style," she replied. "The bridesmaids are all different sizes, and my matron of honor will be seven months pregnant."

Art jumped into the conversation. "Lee, do we have that problem?"

The discussion of bridesmaids' dresses came to an abrupt halt as laughter broke out around the table.

* * *

Our church inaugurated a plan for the congregation to become better acquainted. Once a month we had assigned guests for Sunday dinner.

One Sunday our designated guests were the elderly progenitors of a large extended family in the church. Intimidated by the honor of hosting such a venerated couple, I took special pains with planning the menu and table settings.

As we sat down to eat, I was pleased with the results of my efforts. The yellow tablecloth and tropical flower arrangement and delicious food lent the perfect ambience for getting better acquainted with the gracious couple who had joined us for lunch.

The tempo of the conversation picked up steadily through the meal. At one point the elderly lady was laughing and moving her head animatedly. Behind her was a mirror, and the reflection of the back of her bobbing head caught Art's eye.

"Did you see that chicken?" he said leaning from side to side, trying to look around the matronly figure cross the table. "See that tail? That black thing?"

His agricultural sightings detracted from the goal of the afternoon.

* * *

Christmas vacation had come to an end, and Holly, a freshman in college, was flying out at noon. That morning the dread of parting was our breakfast companion. Holly and I were tearfully trying to choke down our food. Tim, less emotional, was silently sad. Oblivious, Art heroically carried on a one-man conversation.

"I'm going to Africa today," he said with enthusiasm.

He repeated the announcement of his imminent departure every few minutes, varying it with the addition of details.

"I'm going to Africa in a water outfit."

"Last time I didn't take Leah Belle, but this time she's going with me."

"We're going to Africa with a missionary outfit."

"Dear," Art said, looking earnestly at Holly, "I'm going to Africa today. Will you be going with me?"

The thought of Holly sailing off for Africa with her grandpa turned a sad breakfast crew into a jolly group.

There are times, however, when Art's mealtime monologues are exasperating. One evening Art was counting everything on his plate. The pile of peas was a daunting challenge.

"Why don't you just forget counting and eat them?" Tim asked.

Art looked at him with surprise. "Well, if I ate them, I couldn't count them."

* * *

Art and I are usually the only ones home for the noon meal. Eating alone with Mystery Woman causes uncomfortable topics to surface.

"Dear, I don't have any money," Art said after checking all his pockets during lunch one day.

"You don't need money," I said.

"Yes, I do—who's going to pay for this food?" he asked, his voice breaking.

"Your son already paid for it," I said, realizing my current identity was proprietor of a restaurant.

"Bless him," Art replied and went back to eating.

I found my purse, pulled out a few dollars, and unobtrusively stuck them in Art's pocket—a precautionary measure in case the topic would come up again, as it so often did.

During lunch another day Art said, "Where's Leah?"

Oh, no. Not again. This is the topic I dread the most.

"Art," I said, gathering my courage and praying for wisdom. "She—uh—" *Oh, what should I say? Any track can get me in deep water.*

"She died," I finally said, deciding to go for the bare truth.

"Again?" he said, with astonishment. "It seems like I've heard that before."

Hoping to steer the conversation away from that topic, I said, "Art, you have many grandchildren."

"I do?" he asked.

"Yes, and two of your grandsons are missionaries. One is in Germany, and the other is in Papua New Guinea."

"Top of the Beginnings—well, well!" Art said, obviously impressed with his descendants.

Hoping to keep the conversation flowing in a positive direction, I started rambling about menu plans, not because it was of interest to Art or of help to me, but rather to avoid any more uncomfortable subjects.

"I have to think of something for Sunday dinner tomorrow," I said.

Art looked at me forlornly. "Do I have to kill a chicken?" he asked. "I hate killing chickens."

"No, we'll have spaghetti," I said, amazed that confiding in Art had helped me come to such a quick decision.

* * *

One day as Art and I were sitting down to lunch, I had an idea. *No need to talk. We'll listen to music.*

I rummaged around and found a tape of old gospel hymns sung by an excellent choir. Perfect! Art had sung in quartets and choirs most of his life. He would love this.

My idea was pure inspiration. He sat there munching his food and humming along.

Wow—this is great, I thought. *He's enjoying it so much. Why didn't I think of this before? It's so much easier than trying to think up dinner conversation.*

Then the random comments started.

"I think I'm supposed to sing with them today," Art said.

"No, it's just a tape," I answered.

"What day is today?" Art asked.

"It's Thursday," I said. Seeing Art's contemplative look, I decided to ward off potential problems by being more definite. "September twelfth," I added.

"Yes," Art said, pausing to think it over a bit. "Yes, that's the day he told me we were singing."

Then he looked at his watch. "But it's only 12:15, and they're singing. Nobody told me we were singing at noon."

"Art, this is just a tape," I said, as I turned off the tape recorder and popped out the tape. "Look—I can turn them off and take the tape out."

"Oh, put it back—I'm enjoying it," Art said.

I put it in the recorder, pushed the play button, and sat down to eat.

The minute I sat down, Art stood up. Heading for the door, he turned and said, "Where am I supposed to meet them?"

My attempt to sidestep dinner conversation had run amuck—obviously nixing any possibility that my avoidance technique had been inspired.

Caregiver Prayer

Dear God, when reality and delusions clash head-on, remind me that my goal is to calm anxious fears and communicate love and respect rather than to set the record straight. Thank you that you always demonstrate love for me even when my ideas and intentions are misguided. Help me extend that same grace to my loved one today. In Jesus' name I pray. Amen.

Just Between Caregivers
Extending Grace to Your Loved

Erase from your vocabulary—

"I just told you."

"Don't you remember?"

"You already told me that."

Don't ask questions that require recent memory.

Don't: "Hi, Dad. Do you remember who this is?"

Do: "Look, Dad! Sharon came with me today."

Don't: "What did you do today?"

Do: "What a nice shirt you have on! I like the color."

Be willing to talk about the past, but don't insist on accuracy.

One day Art was telling about his adventures in Africa. He mentioned that while standing on the coast of Africa, he could see China.

Rather than saying that was impossible, our son responded, "Wow, Grandpa! You had very good eyes!"

14 ✳ The Edge of the Pool

There's a lovely hotel in the highlands of Guatemala that has always intrigued me. The impos-
ing rock structure beckons weary travelers to a
haven of Old World charm. Glimpses through
the arched entryway reveal a lush courtyard with
fountains, flowering bougainvillea, and gleaming
tile walkways. Numerous brick chimneys poking
from the tile roof conjure up visions of a cozy fire
on a chilly evening.

Although we had driven by the hotel many times, we had never given in to its allure. But with Tim's brother and sister-in-law coming to Guatemala to visit us, the time had come.

We checked into our two hotel rooms in the mid-afternoon. Tim and I were in a room that had an extra bed for Art. Our visitors were a few doors away.

The long drive with its alarming hairpin turns had exhausted us all. The first order of business was a nap. Tim, who had driven the whole way, fell asleep immediately. I was starting to doze off. Art was wide-awake and worried.

"Did I park the car in a good place?" he asked.

"Yes, it's in the garage," I answered groggily and then drifted off again.

"Did I get everything out of the car?" came the worried voice from the other bed once more.

I assured him that he had.

All was silent for a few minutes, but then I heard the creaking of the bed and the shuffling of feet. Art was up and heading for the door.

"Art, where are you going?"

"I—I think I left a dog in the car," he said.

Tim turned over and groaned. It was obvious that our valiant chauffer was not going to get any rest with Art in the room. I found my jacket and Art's sweater and steered him out the door.

As we walked up and down the polished red-tile halls and meandered around the courtyard, Art's travel concerns evaporated. Enthralled with the fountain and the flowers, he wondered if the place were for sale, thinking expansively that if it were, he might buy it.

In one corner of the courtyard, we walked through an archway into a room with soft chairs and a cozy fire. We sat down and chatted about life long ago, about trips to Africa, which probably had not happened the way they were now remembered.

I was surprised when a young man approached us with pen and pad in hand. "What would you like to order?" he asked.

Order? I looked around. I had unwittingly led the pious old man into debauchery: there we were talking about his missionary endeavors in the bar.

* * *

Before dinner the other three joined us, and we went on a family outing—a walk through the village. Our purpose was twofold: to see the sights and to tire Art sufficiently so that he would sleep well in his new location.

It was an error in judgment. The late afternoon sun cast odd and lingering shadows on the cobblestone roads. Industrious merchants, setting up booths for the next day's market, created a confusing kaleidoscope of people, colors, and bustling activity.

We did not realize the effect it had on Art until we were seated in the hotel's grand old dining room. As the brothers and we sisters-in-law calmly perused the menu, Art opened and shut his. He laid it down and picked it up. He opened it again, abruptly closed it, and threw it down onto the table.

"I've got to go help that little girl," he said suddenly, scraping his chair away from the table.

"Dad, it's time to eat," Tim said, calmly patting Art's hand.

"I have to help her," Art repeated insistently. "She's all alone."

Both sons tried reasoning with their father, but it was to no avail.

I had an idea.

"Art, you stay here. I'll go look for her." Then I walked out of the dining room and stood in the courtyard a few minutes before returning to the table.

"She's with her parents—everything is fine," I said, ignoring the questioning looks from my in-laws that registered their misgivings regarding not only Art's mental state but mine as well.

They had reason to wonder. My scheme was totally ineffective. The odd conversation continued.

"She's all alone—I have to help her," he said over and over, frantic to be on his way.

The delicious cuisine, the music wafting from the lively marimba group, the crackling fire in the stone fireplace—all of it was lost to us as we attempted to get through our meal before Art bolted in search of an illusory lass who was torturing his mind.

It was a miserable dinner, and the situation deteriorated even more when we retired to our rooms. All night long, Art was on an endless quest. Up and down from his bed, stumbling around in the dark, he searched for his shoes, his wife, his keys, his little girl, his dog, his car—his life.

In retrospect, I think I know how he felt. As a child, I had an aversion to getting water in my eyes. We never thought of using goggles in those days. In the pool I would squeeze my eyes shut and thrash away, thinking I was swimming. One day, I ventured into the deep end. I was not a strong swimmer, if a swimmer at all, and soon realized that I was in big trouble. I could not find the side of the pool, and I was tiring quickly. Actually, I was within reach of the edge, but I had no way of knowing it. With my eyes tightly closed, inches were miles, because try as I might, I could not find my way. I was hopelessly lost in a wet, dark world, until someone pulled me to safety.

In that idyllic spot, Art had totally lost his bearings. The tiring trip, the unusual surroundings, and the chaotic streets completely disoriented his already-confused mind. Frantic, he thrashed about in a hopelessly confusing world, and our attempts to pull him to reality were futile. All night long he searched for the edge of the pool.

The next morning it was a subdued and weary group who loaded into the car to head to our next location.

Yes, that's what I said: our next location. We had prepaid reservations for a lakeside hotel fifty miles down the road, and we were all dreading it.

Before nightfall, I went in search of some sleep-inducing potion. The local pharmacy had Tylenol PM. I carefully read the label. Art did not have glaucoma or inhibited renal function, and he was well over twelve years old. It might help. At least we would be better prepared than we had been the previous night.

That evening Tim helped Art into his pajamas. Before I had time to administer the medication, Art got into bed, without any coercion or even encouragement, and fell sound asleep. He slept flat on his back all night, not waking even once. The only thing that hampered our sleep was the loud snoring exuding from our weary swimmer who had been lost at sea the night before.

Caregiver Prayer

Dear God, thank you that you are my rock, my sure and steady place in this sea of caregiving. Thank you that even when times are hard and I don't know what to do, you will not leave me to flounder on my own. You have promised never to leave me, to be with me always, and to be my help in times of trouble. In Jesus' name I pray. Amen.

Just Between Caregivers
Caregiver Checklist for Traveling with an Alzheimer's Patient

☐ Discuss your travel plans with the patient's physician, and ask specifically what medication to use should agitation occur. If a prescription medication is recommended, buy it and pack it. It's better to have it and not need it, than to need it and not have it.

☐ Have a plan for reuniting with your patient should you become separated. If your patient is registered with MedicAlert+Safe Return,* you should inform them in advance of your travel itinerary, including contact information for each day.

☐ If you'll be traveling alone with the patient, consider inviting another adult to accompany you.

☐ Pack at least two nightlights—one for the bedroom and one for the bathroom. A flashlight is also helpful.

☐ Plan light travel days. Don't exhaust yourself or your patient.

☐ Avoid loud restaurants and crowds.

*The Alzheimer's Association in alliance with MedicAlert offers the Medic-Alert+Safe Return program for Alzheimer's patients. There is an initial registration fee and an annual renewal fee. Alzheimer's patients can be enrolled by calling 888-572-8566 or going online to <www.medicalert.org/safereturn>.

15 ✳ The Activity Director

The chords of the hymn medley were working up to its finale. It was time.

"Art, would you like a snack?"

During the nine hours that Tim is at work, I shuffle Art between his large-print *Reader's Digest* and the piano, serve meals and snacks, and insist on naptime. Occasionally we run errands, and from time to time Art thinks up his own activities—the hedge people need tending, or some other phantom duty beckons him. My favorite days are the ones when he sits by the window and reads for hours. On those days I call him a model citizen.

But for a long time I struggled with a nagging guilt: should I, his activity director, be doing more to make life interesting for him?

I had heard reports about the adult daycare facilities he went to when he lived with his other children. There they had sing-alongs and crafts, played trivia games, tossed beach balls, and did leg lifts from recliners. They even went on a field trip to a park and had a picnic. Life with me as his activity director seemed awfully mundane by comparison.

I shared my concern with our Thursday night dinner crew, the single teachers from the Christian school.

"Why don't you write out an activity plan, kind of like a lesson plan?" one teacher said.

Of course—what a great idea! I'm a teacher. I know how to write plans.

That night I set to work and came up with an impressive schedule of events.

> Read devotional from *Our Daily Bread*
> Play piano
> Water flowers
> Play simplified Scrabble
> Snack
> Look at family photos
> Walk around the block

Read newspaper

Lunch

The next day I put on my activity director hat and kept Art busy all morning. Feeling rather smug about my accomplishment, I set his lunch in front of him.

He ate heartily. "I don't know why I'm so hungry," he said between bites. "I haven't done anything all day."

It was a deflating moment for the activity director.

* * *

Summer loomed before us, a time when Tim and I had a few months of travel on our work schedule. One thing was certain: the constant change would be too much for someone with dementia. Art could not go with us. That summer he spent two months in a nursing home.

One day we were traveling close to Art's nursing home and stopped by for a visit. The aide at the facility expertly punched in the numbers to open the door into the lockdown unit, explaining the reason for the precaution—patients in this section had flight tendencies.

She directed us to a large room where a number of residents were sitting and said that we would find Art in there. Except for a man in a wheelchair who was ranting and shaking his fist, everyone in the room looked the same. With sagging shoulders and drooping heads, they sat, as though life were a burden. A television set in the corner was airing a soap opera, but no one seemed to be watching. No one was doing anything. I wondered why they were in a lockdown unit. Not one looked capable of taking flight.

On my first perusal, I did not see Art. As my eyes slowly scanned the room a second time, there was something familiar about the silver-haired gentleman slumped on the couch—familiar and yet so foreign.

Could that slouching, rumpled man be Art? Surely not! But it was. Art sat, like all the others, head down with his long chin nearly touching his chest. He had on his favorite pink shirt, but even that had a derelict look to it. The pocket had come loose on one side and was drooping, just like Art.

My activity director mind could not comprehend why he was just sitting, doing nothing. I knew he could sit for hours and read the same page or wind his watch incessantly, but I had never seen him dumbly slumped in a seat, totally inert.

Perhaps it was because he had nothing to do. There was no reading material in the room, and he was not wearing his watch. When I asked about the watch, I was told that the nursing staff was afraid another patient would take it, so they had sent it home with the family.

We went over to him. "Hi, Dad!"

He raised his head and stared oddly, as though we were barely visible, hidden by a fog.

We cajoled him into standing up and going on a walk. His once-sturdy shuffle was tentative and unsteady. He displayed no interest in his surroundings. Not even the enclosed garden that was bursting with a riot of colorful flowers evoked any comment from him.

On that short walk, I realized that hints about characters or plots or settings—clues into Art's novel of the day—were never given there. In that lockdown unit no novels existed. Chemical restraints, given to control his wanderings, had constricted his already-impaired mental processes.

If we had not been planning on taking Art home in a few weeks, the search for another facility would have begun. There are places where those with flight tendencies are allowed to flutter their wings.

But Art returned to our home, and I resumed my role as activity director, no longer plagued by even a twinge of guilt. Art has a wealth of activities—a watch to wind, a large-print *Reader's Digest* to read, a piano to play, and the hedge people to pastor. He's a busy man.

Caregiver Prayer

Dear God, if I should be doing more for my loved one, bless me with specific ideas of what to do and the energy to carry them out. Give me wisdom to reject feelings of inadequacy and guilt that come from my own unrealistic expectations or those of others. May my heart be at peace and my loved one blessed with the care I give today. In Jesus' name I pray. Amen.

16 ✳ The Spirit Is Fine

Art was full of "I hopes" on the midnight flight
from Los Angeles to Guatemala:

"I hope this has enough gas to get us there."

"I hope this stays up until we're supposed to
come down."

"I hope the guy up there knows how to drive
this outfit."

With it being the middle of the night, the other passengers must have had their hopes too—that the old man in aisle 16 would soon go to sleep.

After a while, Art calmed down. He leaned his head back, closed his eyes, and said, "Oh, well, my Savior knows all about it. He'll take care of me."

Art never forgot that God loved him and that he belonged to God. In fact, it was uncanny how confused he could be and yet how right-on he was spiritually.

At church one Sunday morning, a middle-aged woman came up to Art and said, "Would you give me a hug? It's my birthday, and you remind me of my father."

"Is he here?" Art asked.

"No, he's gone," the woman answered, sadly.

"How long?" he said.

"Nine months," she replied.

Art looked at her with tears in his eyes and said, "That's really hard."

They hugged, and she walked away.

A few minutes later, Art was hunting for Leah Belle and asking where he had left his car. He was back chasing his ghosts of the past, but for a fleeting moment of time he had been lucid, full of compassion, and ministering to a woman who missed her father.

Art was a well-educated man with an extensive vocabulary. As dementia progressed, his vocabulary decreased and became muddled.

At breakfast he was staring at his napkin, looking very perplexed. "Do you know what it is?" I asked.

"Yes," he replied, "It's a—a—a beauty mark. Where do you want it?"

When we were out running errands, Art was enthralled with how many cars were on the road. "They're coming in draperies. Oh, here comes a wheel." He pointed at a motorcycle.

But when Art is asked to pray before a meal, he's much more fluent. The words come easier, and his vocabulary is clearer. His prayers are full of praise to his God, who has helped him "these many, many years." His prayers often address the situation precisely, much more than his confused mind could possibly comprehend.

One evening Tim had to work late and would not be home until after Art was in bed. I was feeling sorry for myself. This caregiving was not working out as I had envisioned. I took care of Art all day. Working the swing shift was not on my job description.

When Art and I sat down to dinner, I invited him to ask the blessing. I wasn't up to it.

"Thank you for this food, and thank you for the one who prepared this meal," Art prayed. "Give her joy as she serves others."

Did he know that I was struggling? No, I'm sure he didn't. But God used his prayer to speak to my heart that night.

* * *

A few months later, we had company for dinner, a missionary couple who had worked in Guatemala translating the New Testament for an indigenous group. The New Testament was published and in the hands of the people. The next day that couple was going to board an airplane and leave Guatemala and the people they had served for more than thirty years, to take up new responsibilities in the United States.

That night Tim asked Art to pray before we began eating. We bowed our heads and clasped hands around the table.

"Dear Father, thank you for the food we have today and for how you have helped us these many, many years. Bless these dear ones with us tonight. May their work last and grow. In Jesus' name. Amen."

Art does not know who we are—let alone who our friends were. He was clueless that they were missionaries, leaving their life's work the next day. Yet his prayer echoed the deepest desire of their hearts—that their work would last and grow.

Those were not isolated incidents. It happened over and over. One day a family member asked a medical technician how it could be that Art was so confused and yet prayed so well.

The technician said, "The mind might be gone, but the spirit is fine."

Caregiver Prayer

Dear God, give me insight and creativity into ways I can nourish the spirit as well as meet the physical needs of my loved one today. I confess that I have neglected my own spirit. O God, I need you now as never before. Come and feed my needy heart. In Jesus' name I pray. Amen.

Just Between Caregivers
Cultivating Your Walk with God

When you're a caregiver, nurturing your own spirit is crucial, and it needs to be intentional. Write down the things you're currently doing or could do to cultivate your walk with God. Note the obstacles you're facing and insights the Lord gives you for overcoming them.

_____

_____

_____

_____

_____

_____

_____

The LORD is my shepherd, I shall not be in want.
He makes me lie down in green pastures,
He leads me beside quiet waters,
He restores my soul (Psalm 23:1-3).

17 ✳ The Juggler

In his lifetime Art pastored small and struggling churches, often taking a second job to supplement his income. His jobs varied, but one thing was certain—he was a hardworking man.

For a time Art taught school. His attempt to pursue that career after dementia is legendary in family lore.

Art was living with his daughter in northern California. In an effort to stimulate Art's memory, she gave him a notebook for journaling.

One morning, notebook in hand, Art escaped from the house without being noticed. There was a public high school a few blocks away. Art meandered into the gymnasium and announced to a janitor that he was a substitute teacher reporting for duty. The notebook lent some credibility to his tale. It wasn't long, however, before someone spotted Art's MedicAlert+Safe Return bracelet.

When his daughter arrived to take him home, the old pedagogue was surrounded by a group of people—the janitor, a teacher, and some basketball players—and was lecturing on the wonders of Africa, including anecdotes from his missionary sojourn there. It had been a great day on the job!

Now that Art lives with us, he must find employment within the confines of the hedge. That's no problem. When the need to work arises, there are jobs to do.

I have a number of "someday projects"—tasks that would be nice to do but are not urgent. When I talk about those projects, I often preface the statement with "Someday I'd like to . . . "

"Sand kitchen table" was one of my someday projects. Years ago we bought the table from a family with five children. Between that active tribe and our four kids, the table had received quite a beating. Much of the varnish had worn off, and what little remained was cloudy and opaque. It needed a good sanding before a new waterproof finish could be applied. "Sand kitchen table" was on my someday list for a long time.

One morning when the need to go to an imaginary job was heckling Art, I wrestled the table out to the front lawn. "Someday" had arrived!

Art was by the gate, contemplating the locks.

"Art, I'm so glad you could come to work today. Come with me."

I led him to the table and handed him some sandpaper.

He plunged into the project with the vigor of an employee who knows his boss is watching. This was exhilarating—Art had work, and a someday project was underway.

Tim was also in the front yard that morning, pruning the hedge. I left my worker in his care and made a quick trip to the store.

When I returned, the clippers were propped against an empty ladder standing beside the hedge. On one side of the ladder the top of the hedge was square and straight. On the other side fresh green cypress shoots were poking out at odd angles. The job had been abandoned.

The someday project was still underway. But the industrious worker sanding the table was not Art. Having found an underling to take his place, Art was sitting on a chair in the shade—leaning back, arms crossed like a regular Tom Sawyer, supervising as Tim finished the job.

❋ ❋ ❋

Early one afternoon Art and I were in the car heading home from the store when concerns over potential employment arose.

"Will they have tools?" Art asked.

"Tools?"

"Oh, I should have brought some," he said, taking my hesitation as a no.

He took off his ring and handed it to me. "I better not wear this. I could mess it up."

Mystified, I took the ring.

"Do you know the people I'll be working for?" he asked as we pulled into our driveway.

"Yes," I said, suddenly realizing that Art needed a job.

Before going around to the passenger side, I found the hose and attached it to the spigot. Then I helped Art out of the car, handed him the nozzle, and said, "Water the flowers, please."

I left the industrious workman squirting the flower beds and went into the house.

It wasn't long until I heard the neighbor's pit bull barking furiously. Running outside, I found Art squirting the leaping beast through the fence. The possibility of such a benign job becoming life-threatening had never entered my mind. I ran to the faucet and turned it off with trembling hands.

"That's enough—time for a rest," I said.

Leading Art into the safety of the house, I took him directly to the door that bears the sign "This room belongs to Art Carey."

He stopped and read the poster with astonishment. He had his own resting place on the job! Pleased with such royal treatment, the hired man stretched out on the bed with a sigh and fell asleep.

But the old dear is still juggling secondary jobs with his true vocation. When he awoke, his pastoral duties were calling him. He hurried about looking for his tie, checking his watch. He was anxious to be on time for his next responsibility.

Caregiver's Prayer

Dear God, I'm a juggler too—juggling caregiving with all my other responsibilities. Give me a keen eye to see what my priorities should be each day, grace to handle the unexpected, and peace in my heart. Grant me wisdom to know when I'm juggling too much and courage to cut back, even if I have to eliminate things that in themselves are good.

Just Between Caregivers:
Evaluating the Load You're Carrying

Even the best juggler has a limit to how many balls he or she can keep in the air. You have your limits too.

In our early days in Guatemala, we had no refrigerator. Every morning I walked to the market to buy the day's ration of food. One day I headed out with a basket on my arm and a baby on my back. At the market I bought a hunk of meat, a few potatoes, some carrots, and an onion. *That would make a nice stew.* One of the sellers had fresh pineapples. *Perfect for dessert!* I bought a big one. My basket was full to overflowing, weighing heavily on my arm. But just as I was leaving the market, I spotted a rare treasure—a watermelon! It was such an incredible find that I couldn't pass it up, so I bought it. Our house was uphill from the market. By the time I had reached home with my heavy load, my arms were quivering, my legs were weak, and I was nauseous.

Nothing I bought was bad. On the contrary, the pineapple was golden and sweet; the watermelon was crisp and juicy. No, it was not the individual items but rather the combined weight of all those good things that made me sick from exhaustion.

During this season of life some activities or responsibilities —even good things—may need to be suspended so that you can juggle with greater ease the caregiving task God has placed in your hands.

18 ✳ Something Seems Suspicious

In the English language, the pronouns *they* and *them* are sometimes used to indicate a vague group of people—not a group in which you could name each individual, but rather an unidentifiable group. That unidentifiable group comes to haunt us from time to time.

One afternoon when I thought Art was napping, I found him creeping stealthily through the living room.

"Sh-h-h," he said, holding his forefinger to his lips.

In guarded whispers, he informed me that we had to do something. *They* were coming to steal our things.

"We're the only ones in the house," I told him, "and the gate is locked. We're safe."

No, he was quite sure we were in danger of being robbed.

He pointed to a picture over the piano—an oil painting of a cottage on rolling hills done in pastel colors.

"*They're* in there," Art whispered.

"Oh," I said, at a loss for a more apt response to such a revelation.

We stood there staring at the picture.

"Aren't you going to do something?" Art said.

"Yes," I said, motioning for him to follow me.

We tiptoed out to the kitchen and shut the swinging door, putting a barrier between us and *them*. Then I gave Art a large bowl of ice cream, adding the distance of a sweet distraction between us and *them*.

Somewhere in that cold, creamy substance, Art's worries about thieves lurking in a pink cottage over the piano melted away.

* * *

At four-thirty one Sunday morning, *they* were back. Tim found Art wandering through the house looking for *them*.

That morning, putting Art back to bed was like punching the snooze button on an alarm clock. Every few minutes he was up again. He thought someone was in the house and up to no good.

Getting more sleep was a losing battle, so we got up. I made some coffee. Tim turned on the shower and informed Art it was time to bathe.

No, Art did not want a shower. Now that we were up and dressed for the day, he was tired and wanted to go to bed.

After tucking his dad in for the tenth time that morning, Tim went for a run. There's nothing like vigorous exercise to relieve frustration.

It wasn't long until I heard the tell-tale shuffle, shuffle, shuffle. It was Art, of course, looking for *them*. I turned on all the lights in the house to eliminate any dark corners where *they* could be hiding.

"Come have a cup of coffee, and we'll decide what to do about *them*," I said.

He sat at the little breakfast table in his red pajamas, sipping his coffee with his thin white hair sticking out in all directions.

After a while he said, "I think I've scared *them* off."

I couldn't help but laugh.

"Yes, anyone seeing you in those red pajamas would be scared to death," I said. And Art laughed too.

* * *

One afternoon Art was extremely tired, walking all bent over like a flag flying at half-mast. I put him down for a nap, but he kept getting up. I should have just given in to the inevitable, but I did not want Tim to come home and find his father so worn out. With that noble goal in mind, I was insistent—escorting Art back to bed each time he got up.

It was no use. He never slept. Finally, when I heard him rummaging around in the closet in his room, I went in and asked if he would like a snack.

"Sh-h-h," he whispered. "Be quiet. *They* won't let me out of here."

Fortunately, he did not remember that I was the unidentifiable *they* holding him captive.

* * *

One evening, Holly, Art, and I went shopping and returned home as the sun was setting. The last vestiges of sunlight cast an eerie glow into the nearly dark house as we entered. In that spooky entrance, *they* came to haunt us.

I flipped on the light and helped Art take off his jacket.

"When will *they* be home?" he said with concern in his voice.

"I don't know," I replied, thinking perhaps he meant Tim, who would be coming home quite late because of a meeting.

All evening, Art worried about *them*—not that *they* would cause us trouble but rather that we were causing problems for *them*.

At dinner he gave the blessing and included a plea for *them*. "Help us to be able to see *them* soon. Lord, you can do anything, so help *them* to come soon."

During the meal, the topic of whether *they* wanted us in *their* home and where *they* might be came up frequently.

He was still worried about our brazen act of breaking and entering when I was tucking him in bed. This was such a lovely home, and *they* were not here.

"Dear, what is *their* name?"

When I told him that *they*—the owners—were named Carey, he nestled down in his covers with a sigh of relief.

"Well, well," he said, reassured that the unidentifiable group bore the family name. "Maybe *they* won't mind."

Caregiver's Prayer

Dear God, you know what is hidden in darkness, and light dwells with you. When doubts and suspicions trouble the mind of my dear one, shine your light on the situation. You are the God of peace. Please bring your peace to our hearts and our home, even when things seem suspicious.

19 ❋ The Sweepstakes

Tim and I are not alone in our journey as caregivers. A number of our friends are also caring for a parent or spouse with dementia. Although our caregiving situations are unique and the causes of dementia vary, there is one common thread—we all face challenges.

Sharon, one of our single friends, closed up her house and moved from one side of the United States to the other to join forces with her sister in the care of their mother. Because of that move, Sharon became a member of "Friday Ladies."

This is a group of elderly women who meet on Friday mornings to prepare craft materials for the 200 preschoolers who attend Sunday School at their church. Sharon's mother has been a member of the Friday Ladies for years. She can no longer do the counting or sorting jobs, but she can still cut out handwork pieces and enjoys being with the other women. Her days of attending alone have passed, so Sharon goes with her.

One Friday morning Sharon's mom needed to use the restroom. The Friday Ladies meet in the children's education wing of the church, and the girls' bathroom has four stalls. The farthest from the door is handicap accessible, but the other three are narrow stalls designed for children and have lower toilets.

In a hurry, her mother chose the stall closest to the door. The dear woman is nearly silent these days, so Sharon was surprised when she heard a soft cry for help coming from the stall. With a series of yes/no questions, she determined that her mother was stuck on the toilet and could not open the door.

When I was in elementary school, locking the stall door and then crawling out was a common prank. When the deed was discovered, the teacher would send a responsible, lithe volunteer under the door to open it.

Having been a teacher, Sharon knew the protocol, but there were no small volunteers to come to the rescue. Sharon is a large woman—not fat but quite solid and tall, and it was up to her to get that door open. After all, at sixty years old, she was the youngest member of the Friday Ladies group.

Down on her stomach, the caregiver warrior inched her way into the stall with her elbows, flattening herself as closely to the floor as she could while she slithered under the partition.

Once inside, the battle was not over. The cramped space, older knees, twenty extra pounds, and the obstacle of another adult sitting on the toilet were all hindrances to maneuvering into an upright position. Like an inchworm, she scrunched to a hands-and-knees position and, balancing on one hand, used the other to open the door. With much grappling, she was able to stand and then helped her mother off the toilet.

Mission accomplished, the valiant caregiver and her mother returned, arm in arm, to resume their Friday Ladies duties in the project room.

❊ ❊ ❊

Another of our caregiving friends is a professor—a quiet, dignified, and respected man. He and his wife are caring for his elderly father, who is fixated on winning the sweepstakes.

His fascination began years ago. No longer able to drive, the old gentleman remembered with fondness the years after his retirement when he and his wife toured the United States with their Airstream travel trailer. Those had been the best years of his life.

Driven by a craving for renewed independence and mobility, he became enthralled with the sweepstakes offers that arrived in his mailbox. With that much money, he could a buy a new Airstream and a vehicle to pull it, and even hire a chauffer to take him on another See America tour.

The sweepstakes fliers were written by gifted authors—true craftsmen in their trade. While carefully avoiding the outright declaration that the recipient had won or was about to win, they left the distinct impression that this was the final cut and that the odds for winning were great. The professor's father believed that a quick response would likely result in big money and the realization of his dream.

The entry forms often had stickers to attach or questions to answer in a precise way. Entering was a complex business, so the old fellow enlisted the professor as his personal sweepstakes secretary.

The professor is a good man, honest to the core. He had always related to his father in a factual and rational way, so after meticulously filling out the entry forms under his father's watchful eye, he faithfully mailed each and every one. He promised he would, so he did.

The father cajoled his son into supplying him with the latest Airstream catalogues and vehicle brochures and then sat for hours in his recliner, pad and pencil in hand, plotting how he would spend his sweepstakes money.

Knowing his father's dream was illogical, the professor tried to bring reason to the situation. He researched and found statistics to share with his father on the dismal chances of ever winning the sweepstakes. When the elderly gentleman wanted to order products from brochures that accompanied the sweepstakes offers, he showed him the fine print that said no purchase was necessary. When his father continued to insist that a purchase would enhance his chances, the professor assisted him in choosing good books or useful household items.

The professor tried his best, but as the years progressed, his father became delusional, and winning the sweepstakes became an outright obsession.

One of the delusions was regarding television. Assisted by hired caregivers in an apartment attached to the professor's house, the father refused to let the caregiver undress him if the television set was on. It was improper—the people on television would see him. He not only thought they could see him but also was convinced that they could interact with him.

One day the elderly gentleman, with a sweepstakes coupon in his hand, dozed off in his recliner while watching television. Half asleep and half awake, he thought he heard his name.

His name! The people on television were calling his name! His moment had come! He had won the sweepstakes! He had to show them his number.

The old gentleman fell trying to get to the television set, cut his head, and had to have stitches.

A few weeks later, the delusion happened again, and the professor received a frantic call from the caregiver.

Running to the apartment, he found his ancient father hovering precariously in front of the television with his sweepstakes coupon in hand. He refused to sit down until his winning status was acknowledged by a television personage.

The professor, who always related to his father in a rational way, acted true to form. He reasoned with him and finally convinced the determined old gentleman to sit down.

But the negotiation was a compromise in logic. Handing the remote to the hired man with instructions to flip through the channels, the professor stationed himself in front of the television set. As giraffes loped across an African landscape on the Discovery Channel, a battle was fought on the History Channel, and a CNN special showed life in an impoverished country, the dignified professor held the piece of paper in front of the screen and waited—for either an acknowledgement of the winnings or his father to fall asleep.

Caregiver Prayer
Dear God, today I pray for the many others who are caregivers, beginning with those of my own family who are facing this challenge

with me. May the pressure of caregiving draw us together rather than push us apart. Help us to be a team who works together, trusts one another, and cheers each other on.

I also pray for my friends, near and far, who are caregivers. May they feel your strengthening power lifting them up today. Give them wisdom for each difficult situation, courage to face the uncertainties ahead, peace in perplexities, and joy when they least expect it. In Jesus' name I pray. Amen.

Just Between Caregivers
Upholding Each Other

Comrades in arms, fellow soldiers in this battle of caregiving, somehow it helps to share our predicaments with people who have been in similar circumstances.

While some situations are humorous and fun to share, others are not. My friend's mother became paranoid. She was sure her daughter was out to get her money and was stealing things from her. Not wanting to defame her mother nor be a complainer, my friend shared with no one the burden she was bearing. The hurt dug its way deep into her heart, and she bore it alone for months. Finally she had a long talk with her sister. They became allies in the battle rather than pawns pitted against each other. She also found support in a small group of friends who meet together weekly to pray. As comrades in the challenges of life, her friends pray for her, even when she's too weary or upset to pray for herself.

Make a list of the caregivers you know, and list the challenges they're facing. If you don't know their challenges, ask. Pray for those friends, and ask them to pray for you.

_____

_____

_____

_____

_____

_____

_____

_____

P. S. Before you attempt a belly crawl to rescue your loved one from a bathroom stall, check the lock on the outside of the door. Yes, it's usually just a flat, stainless steel circle, but the center of that circle sometimes has a groove. Inserting the edge of a quarter into that groove and turning it can open the lock.

20 ✳ Home Alone

Art and I stood by the gate and waved goodbye to Tim. Work was calling him to the hinterlands of Guatemala. For a few days it was going to be just the two of us facing life's challenges together. I hoped they would not be many.

I had already decided to sidestep one issue. While his valet was traveling, Art was going to have a reprieve from bathing.

The next morning, however, I was awakened by the sound of running water. It was Art. He was showering at 5:30 A.M. How is it that when Tim wants him to bathe, it takes some coaxing to get him going, but when I don't want him to, there he is showering before dawn?

Art is a thorough bather. He scrubs up and rinses off. Then, forgetting that he's already done it, he scrubs up again and again and again. That morning he was in the shower a very long time.

"Art," I said through the bathroom door, "is everything going all right?"

"Yes, I have one foot soaped up," he reported, "and now I'm doing the other one. But it's r-e-a-l-l-y slippery."

"Art, don't worry about your feet—just rinse off and get out," I said with alarming visions of a fall and broken hip racing through my mind.

He finally emerged from the bathroom carrying the fluffy green bathmat—wondering if he was supposed to wear it or take it.

I hustled him into the bedroom and helped him dress in more appropriate attire.

In the morning mail we received a calendar with pictures of Papua New Guinea from our son.

"Art, look what your grandson sent us," I said.

Art was enthralled. He looked through it as if he had just received a family picture album.

"Here's Leah Belle," he said, pointing to the January page with a group of natives coming home from fishing.

He was sure that the fierce, dark-skinned warrior with white face paint on the July page was his dad.

"Whooee!" Art said as he flipped to October and showed me his relatives—some dancers decked out in little more than paint and leaves.

That afternoon Art was hoping to get his picture in the family album too. He was walking around the house, standing a little straighter, smiling and looking around expectantly.

When he passed by me the third time, he said, "Do you think they got my picture yet? I've been walking around and think they might have gotten it."

That night as I tucked Art into bed, he said, "Dear, if you hear anything in the night, you'd better check. It might be me. I might be up to something."

It was a vain threat. We had an uneventful night. The next morning I got up early, hoping to forestall any impromptu bathing.

I peeked into Art's room to see if he was awake. He was, but he was still in bed, all bundled up in his covers, a good place to be on a chilly morning.

As I was turning to go, I heard a puffing sound. Looking again, I saw Art blowing under his covers.

I was curious. "What are you doing?" I asked.

"Giving them air," he said.

"Who?"

"The people under the covers. They need air. Wouldn't you need air if you were under there?"

"You're the only one in the bed," I said.

"Are you sure?" he asked.

Even though I was sure, Art was not. He stayed in bed a while longer, periodically puffing under the covers to keep his illusory visitors from asphyxiating.

The next morning we had real visitors—two women from our church. They had heard Tim was traveling and were concerned that I might be lonely.

I ushered them and Art into the dining room and served lemonade and cookies. The ladies are sisters, and it didn't take much to induce them to tell stories of how they and the others in their clan met their spouses.

In the midst of an episode, one of the matrons stopped mid-sentence and said, "Art, why aren't you drinking your lemonade?"

"I'm too busy looking at you ladies," he replied. "I can't decide who's the prettiest."

Judging by the titters and blushing smiles, it had been a long time since those matriarchs had perplexed a man in that way.

After lunch I found the old charmer hunkered down on the couch with his *Reader's Digest*.

"Wouldn't you like to sit over here? The light is better," I said, indicating a chair by the window where he usually sat to read.

No, he did not. There were a lot of people out there who wanted something for nothing, and he did not want to be seen.

"Time for a nap," I said.

"Nap?" he said indignantly. "Nap, nip, nope. They put them in rows for us, but they still let us sing. All they want is our money."

Having said that, he walked over to the piano in full view of the hedge people and played a few lively tunes. Then he sauntered off to his room with no assistance, got into bed, and took a long nap.

I was making dinner when he got up and didn't notice when he came into the kitchen.

"Ahem."

I turned around when I heard him clear his throat. "Well, Art, what are you doing?"

He stood by the table, hands clasped behind his back, smiling shyly. "Oh, just standing here, hoping."

"Hoping for what?"

"Breakfast."

Art was hungry, and the food was ready, so we sat down to an early supper.

As we ate, I was silently reflecting on how well Art had adjusted to being home alone with me. At that moment he leaned over and gave me his evaluation.

In a confidential whisper he said, "Dear, this place is crazy. Everyone here is just a little crazy. But I've gotten used to it."

Caregiver Prayer

Dear God, it's true! Life can be a little crazy in my role as caregiver. When life's changing scenes require extra duty, be my strength and help. Give me joy for the task and enough respite to maintain perspective. In Jesus' name I pray. Amen.

21 ✳ It Seemed So Harmless

I found Art talking to an elderly gentleman one day. Art was telling him the names of his seven children, counting them off on his fingers. The old man listened with head bowed, counting the children on his fingers too. Then he looked up, just as Art looked up. Art was proud that he had listed them all. The man beamed at him. He was impressed.

Encouraged, Art chuckled, and the man chuckled with him. He shifted from one foot to another, and the old fellow shifted too. What a pair! They were having a great time—Art talking, and the kind, old gentleman listening with such rapt attention that his mouth moved to Art's every word.

"It's time to go, Art," I called.

He waved good-bye, and the silver-haired gentleman waved back.

"That's my friend," he said. "He's a Carey."

Yes, he was a Carey—he was Art Carey's own reflection in the mirror.

Art's bedroom was directly across the hall from Holly's room, which has a full-length mirror facing the door. From time to time Art would spot his friend as he walked past her room and go in for a chat. One afternoon he spent an entire hour telling the man in the mirror of days gone by and of his large family. The man in the mirror had such patience with Art's repetitive monologue. I left the door open. Their friendship seemed harmless.

Harmless, that is, until the day Art invited the man in the mirror to come in and sit down. Moving toward the bedroom door, Art motioned for his friend to follow him, but his friend did not come. Art was insistent. He walked closer to his friend, and his friend walked closer to him. Art reached out his hand, and his friend extended his hand. Art's hand hit the mirror. Confused, he reached out again and again. Each time, he touched cold glass instead of the warm, extended hand of his friend.

Art walked determinedly outside. He would get his friend and bring him in another door. He tromped all the way around the house but could not find him. He went back to the mirror. Indeed! His friend was still there.

He became obsessed with the desire to bring his friend inside. He tried to pull him from the mirror, but he could not reach him. He went outside, but he could not find him. In and out he went, becoming more agitated all the time. There had to be a way to get to his friend.

"Art, it's time for lunch," I called, but he would not come unless his friend came with him.

I shut our daughter's door, but he came right back to it.

"My friend is in there," Art said.

"No one is in there," I said with the conviction of one who knows the truth.

Art flung open the door and proved me wrong. There he was!

The frantic search, the quest to pull his friend from the mirror, the frenzied pace went on and on. The minutes became hours, or did they only seem like hours because of their intensity?

I could stand it no more. Art was outside searching. I grabbed my purse, locked the house, and opened the car door.

"Art, get in. We must go. It's an emergency."

He looked at me reproachfully, "You don't care about my friend."

"It's an emergency. Get in the car. We must go."

Yes, we *must* go. We must get away.

My leg was shaking as I pushed in the clutch. Hand trembling, I turned the key in the ignition. As one escaping from imminent danger, I threw the car in reverse and tore out of the driveway. We roared away in silence. Art was bewildered, and I was intent on our escape. My only destination was *away*.

Away from what? I pondered as we wove our way through the busy city traffic a half hour later. *Away from the man in the mirror? He didn't exist unless Art was there.*

I was escaping, and yet the main culprit was sitting right next to me in the car.

I glanced over at Art. He looked like a model citizen now, calmly gazing out the window at the bustling world around us.

I knew in that moment that the obsession had faded and that Art was fine, but I did not turn around and go home. We stayed out all afternoon—stopping for an ice cream cone, walking through the grocery store—anything but going home. Art might have forgotten, but I had not. That innocent friendship had turned into something monstrous, and one doesn't recover quickly after seeing a monster.

Caregiver's Prayer

Dear God, what will the next surprise be? Help me face the future with courage and good cheer, even the unknowns of this disease, fully assured that you are with me—today, tomorrow, and always.

22 ✳ Getting It All Together

Thanksgiving Day! Perhaps it was the aroma of the turkey baking in the oven that inspired Art's hasty travel plans on Thanksgiving morning. He was intent on heading out to California. But a trip is hard to pull off without some necessary items. Where was his car? Where were his keys? Traveling is a complicated matter when those things are missing.

My busy morning of Thanksgiving preparations was frequently interrupted by Art, who was urgently trying to get everything together for his trip. The keys and the car were the most-mentioned necessities, but there were other things that would be helpful.

He went into his bedroom, pulled out an odd assortment of clothes, and rolled them up. He stuffed little things from around the house into his shirt pocket such as loose change, a daily verse reminder, an old letter, a sponge from the bathroom. Oh, my—there was so much to take! Then he was back in the kitchen, with his bulky roll of clothes under his arm and shirt pocket bulging. "Have you seen the box with a handle to put these in?" he asked.

"Art, today is Thanksgiving. Why don't you postpone your trip until tomorrow?"

"No, I need to go now. But—" he said with a hopeful look on his face, "a box of eats would be nice. Have you seen my car?"

As the morning progressed, the search became more frantic. He needed to be on his way, but his car and keys were nowhere to be found. He stopped his hunt only for a few minutes to grab a bite of lunch, and then he was off looking again.

By early afternoon I was so weary of his relentless searching and so desperate to be left in peace to finish pulling together Thanksgiving dinner that I took the old preacher by the hand and said, "We're going to pray about your problem. You pray first."

Art prayed that he would find his things and be on his way.

I prayed that he would know the truth and that the truth would set him free.

When we finished praying, Art looked up and said, "Have you seen my car?"

"What color is it?" I asked, knowing full well he had no car.

"It's—it's—I don't know," he answered. "Have you seen it?"

"What kind is it?" I asked. "Is it a Ford?"

"Yes, it's a Ford. No, wait—it's not a Ford. It's a—a—I don't know what it is," he finally concluded, hanging his head.

By then, he was exhausted by his endless hunt and allowed me to lead him to his bed. I took off his shoes and covered him up. And he slept.

When he awakened, he was no longer a traveling man. Instead, he was a very mellow school teacher, content to sit in the living room surrounded by his imaginary students. From what I could hear from the kitchen, it sounded as if the class were taking dictation from Art's reading of the cover of a large-print *Reader's Digest*. They had written "Large Print" many, many times and had finally gotten to "Digest." As I was opening the door for our Thanksgiving guests, I overheard the sage old teacher say, "Digest—when anybody digests, that means they've got it all together."

Caregiver's Prayer

Dear God, help me remember that caregiving takes time. Help me pace myself and schedule my days lightly so that I won't be overwhelmed when life here takes an odd turn.

23 ✳ A Calculated Risk

"What?" I asked, quite sure that I hadn't heard right.

"Dad is going to accompany my solo at the Christmas Eve service," Tim repeated with a hint of pride in his voice. "'Hark! the Herald Angels Sing.'"

I was worried. It's not that Art can't play the piano. He can. Actually, he's quite good. I enjoy his distinctive style—the rich chords and fancy runs that he learned as a child on a player piano. But because of dementia, his mind strays, and he plays snatches of hymns and choruses—one flowing into another—medleys of sorts. The medleys vary but inevitably end with a rousing, syncopated rendition of Bill Gaither's famous song "He Touched Me."

As long as Tim was willing to sing a "Hark! the Herald Angels Sing"/"He Touched Me" medley, it might work. But then again, there could be other problems that would be impossible to predict.

* * *

One afternoon as Art was playing the piano, the tempo of his hymn medley became faster and faster, and he finished with a triumphant flourish, crying out, "I beat him!"

"Beat whom?" I asked.

"Him!" Art responded. "See? He's right here." He pointed to the inside of the lamp on top of the piano. "Max! Max is his name, and he's a big one."

I got up to look at his competitor. There inside the lampshade was a little sticker that read "MAX 60 WATTS."

What will Tim do if Art spies Max during "Hark! the Herald Angels Sing"? Can he sing that fast? Worse yet, what if Art is hyperfocused on Christmas Eve?

One day Art was focused on his watch. He wound his battery-operated watch for over an hour. Unconvinced that it was keeping time, he kept asking what time it was. Trying to divert his focus, I persuaded him to play a song for me.

He sat down at the piano and stared at the keys. "I don't get it," he said. "What time is it?"

"Five-ten," I answered.

He counted out five keys and put a finger on the fifth and then counted five more to make ten. He played the two keys as a chord but shook his head, unsatisfied that 5:10 sounded right.

"What time is it?" he asked again.

He never did get around to playing anything that evening.

Then there was the occasion when he thought the piano was full of people and was trying to get them out. It wasn't a very musical situation.

With experiences like that, it's no wonder I was skeptical when Tim told me that he was going to have Art accompany him at the Christmas Eve service. Art was a talented pianist, but we never knew when he would get off on a tangent or another song.

* * *

About a week before Christmas, the practicing started in earnest. Tim asked Art to play "Hark! the Herald Angels Sing." Art started with that carol, but before he got to the chorus, he switched to "Silent Night." He played only half of that before his mind took him down the irresistible funnel of "He Touched Me." In other practice sessions Tim sang, and that helped Art stay on the right tune, but he stumbled through the song rather miserably. One thing I have to say for my husband is that he's a determined man and not one to give up in the face of unbeatable odds.

Christmas Eve came, and the church was packed. Tim guided Art up to the piano. Then he took the microphone and told the congregation how thankful he was for a church where our children played their first musical pieces and everyone was supportive. He thanked them for allowing Art to play in the twilight years of his life.

Many what-ifs were whirling around in my mind as Tim leaned over and asked Art to start playing "Hark! the Herald Angels Sing."

"I can't," Art whispered, unable to remember the tune.

"That's okay—just give me an F chord, and I'll sing it by myself," Tim whispered back.

Art started Tim off in the Key of G, testing the upper limits of his tenor range. It wasn't going well.

But then an amazing thing happened. As Tim sang the first line, Art began to pick out the melody with one finger. Then he progressed to playing a few chords, hesitantly at first, but eventually working into his full player piano style. He stayed with "Hark! the Herald Angels Sing" through all the verses, not veering off to another tune even once. It went perfectly—belying every doubt I had had.

The final "Glory to the newborn King" still hung in the air as the crowd burst into applause. Art had done an extraordinary job, despite dementia. There were tears glistening in many eyes that night as the talented old pianist and his son walked arm in arm back to their seats. It was a grand finale for Art's closing performance—and his last Christmas.

Caregiver's Prayer

Dear God, give me courage to seek ways for my loved one to participate in life as fully as possible. Put us with gracious people who will accept the limitations we face and cheer even failed attempts.

24 ✳ The Final Launch

Art was a healthy man, even in his nineties. It
seemed that he would be one of those rare indi-
viduals who would pass the one-hundred-year
mark and just keep on going.

In his ninety-fifth year, Art underwent a minor surgical procedure. When the anesthesiologist connected him to various monitors in the operating room, he thought that perhaps one was not functioning properly, because Art's readings were too good for a man his age. He disconnected it from Art and connected himself. The anesthesiologist and the surgeon started laughing. Art's stats were better than his.

Yes, Art was healthy in body, and I had visions of being an elderly woman still taking care of him. But it was not to be.

In his ninety-sixth year, Art's bone marrow stopped producing blood cells. The man who before could tromp out to the hedge several times a day became too weak to walk from one room to another. We commandeered the rolling chair from the office to move him from place to place.

One afternoon Art was tired. I pushed him into his room and with great effort moved him from the office chair to his bed. He was so weak, and the chair, of course, had no brakes—the makings for a precarious transfer at best.

Awhile later, I peeked in to see if he was sleeping. He was, but not in bed. He was in the office chair! There he sat with his feet propped up on the bed and his hands clasped behind his head, like an executive taking a snooze at his desk.

How that feeble man ever got into such a position without breaking his neck I'll never know. But I did know one thing—I would never again leave Art and the rolling office chair in the same room unattended.

As the days passed, Art was in bed more than he was up. We no longer dressed him for the day but rather changed his pajamas each time we bathed him. His appetite dwindled. I bought a few jars of baby food—fruit compotes—to see if he would find them palatable. He was not very interested.

A friend let us borrow a wheelchair. Even with that, I could no longer safely take care of him by myself. Tim began working from home so he would be available to help when needed.

It seemed that the end was near—so much so that Tim asked a men's quartet from our church if they would prepare a few numbers to sing at Art's imminent funeral.

Then Art had one terrible week. First, he had a five-hour ordeal in the emergency room with a bowel impaction. Two days later he passed a kidney stone. Two days after that, he suffered a stroke.

The stroke occurred in the morning. Art was sitting on the edge of his bed, and Tim was buttoning his clean pajama top. All of a sudden, Art started listing to the right. His speech was garbled. His right arm and his right leg were completely paralyzed.

We called our family physician. He told us to do two things: try to get Art to drink so that his swallowing mechanism would continue to function, and start giving him a medication right away.

It was a difficult day. Art could not remember that he was paralyzed. He would try to get up, but could not. He was obviously frustrated, but because of the loss of speech, he could not vocalize his frustration.

Once when I checked on Art I was surprised to see that he was doing his own sort of physical therapy. With his good left hand, he was moving the fingers on his paralyzed right hand. Oddly, each time he moved a finger, the corresponding toe on his right foot also moved.

At five in the afternoon Tim went to do an errand. I was home alone with Art, who lay paralyzed in his bed. I was on the couch reading when I heard a sound in the hall. Shuffle, shuffle,

shuffle. I turned my head to see what it was, and the book fell from my hands.

It was Art, walking out of the bedroom unassisted. He had not been walking by himself even before the stroke. How could he be walking now? It was like seeing Lazarus come forth from the tomb.

After that, the wheelchair started collecting dust. Art was stronger and walking again. He wanted to get dressed in regular clothes, and his appetite increased.

One night the phone rang while we were eating dinner. It was one of the men from the quartet. They were at the church practicing and wanted to consult Tim on the selections to be sung at Art's funeral.

Art's funeral?

What was wrong with this picture?

The man for whose funeral they were preparing was sitting at the table fully dressed, eating meatloaf and potatoes.

* * *

Three weeks later, Art was on the couch reading. When the drone of his voice stopped, I looked up and saw him gazing at the ceiling—his face alight with joy and wonder.

"Art, do you see something?" I asked.

"Yes," he said. "My people."

Curious, I went and sat beside him and looked intently at the same spot on the ceiling. I saw nothing but the tongue-in-groove boards and varnished rafters.

"Do you know their names?" I asked, still staring at the ceiling.

"The ones who tell about Jesus," he said as he smiled up at them.

Heaven is the dwelling place of those who believe in Jesus. That night, heaven seemed a little closer, more real than ever before.

Art lived two weeks longer. Then one day his breathing became labored, and by afternoon it was obvious that he was dying. Tim sat by his bed and sang hymns.

At one point Art struggled to sit up. He asked two questions. The first was garbled and unintelligible. Tim tried to reassure his father and help him lie down. But Art was not done. He made a large sweeping motion with his arm as though he saw a great multitude before him and gasped, "Who will tell all of these about the Lord?"

"With the help of many others, I will," Tim said. "We'll do what we can to see that they have a chance to hear."

Satisfied, Art lay down, never to speak again. Three hours later, he entered the wonders of heaven.

❋ ❋ ❋

The hedge still surrounds our yard—a constant reminder of Art and his years with us. Looking back, we would not trade those years for easier, less challenging ones. It was a time of reciprocal blessing. We honored our father by caring for him when he could no longer care for himself, and in his final launch, he enlarged our vision of heaven and clarified our mission on earth.

Caregiver's Prayer

Dear God, as I see the decline of my loved one and deal with the daily frustration it causes, lift my sight above the challenges of today and comfort me with the eternal hope you have for us. Dementia and physical suffering will not exist in your everlasting kingdom. Thank you for your magnificent promise that one day you will make every-

thing new. Give me courage to face whatever may come today with joyful hope in honor of you.

> *God himself will be with them and be their God.*
> *He will wipe every tear from their eyes.*
> *There will be no more death or mourning or crying or pain,*
> *for the old order of things has passed away.*
> *He who was seated on the throne said,*
> *"I am making everything new!"* (Revelation 21:3-5).

Epilogue

The Things He Never Forgot

A Tribute to My Father-in-Law

Dementia robbed Art of many things—his independence, his sense of time and place, his extensive vocabulary, and the ability to recognize his loved ones. But there were some things so ingrained, so deep inside him, that they endured beyond dementia.

He never forgot—

His wife. Art and Leah Belle were married more than sixty-six years. She preceded him in death by four years, but she never died in his mind. He was sure she was alive and needed him. He spent hours searching for her. A young lady visiting in our home, after a few days of observing Art's undying efforts to find Leah Belle, said she hoped someday to find a man who was that committed to her.

His children. Even though Art got to the point that he did not recognize his children, he repeated their names—in birth order—over and over. He counted them out on his fingers, making sure he had not missed any of the seven. He never forgot them.

To be a gentleman. Art was unfailingly kind and gentlemanly. Even when he was weak and needed help to climb the three stairs into our home, he would invariably step to the side when the door was opened and say with a courtly bow, "Ladies first."

To enjoy life. Art and Leah spent three years in Africa as dorm parents for the children of missionaries serving in the Central African Republic. He loved to tell about his time there. He enjoyed it, as he had all the other things he had done in his lifetime. It's a true gift to be content and to enjoy whatever life brings. In his rambling accounts of experiences real and imagined, of years gone by, Art always ended by saying, "And I enjoyed it."

His relationship with God. Art never forgot that God loved him and that he loved God. He knew God was taking care of him. His prayers at meals were filled with praise and gratitude to the God who had helped him "these many, many years." It was uncanny how confused he could be and yet how right-on his prayers were. Near the end of his life, taking care of him became increasingly difficult. Although he was unaware we were struggling, he prayed many times that God would give his "dear ones" endurance. Art's spirit was fine in spite of dementia.

His passion for the lost to know his Savior. Even on the day he died, Art was concerned for the lost. As noted earlier, his last coherent sentence was "Who will tell all of these about the Lord?"

How to play the piano. Playing the piano was a skill that provided Art with hours of personal enjoyment. Even when dementia had robbed him of so much, he could still play the piano and play it well. If someone sang along, he could stay on a hymn clear to the end. But left on his own, he played snatches of hymns and choruses—one flowing into another—medleys of sorts. His medleys varied, but they always ended with a rousing rendition of the chorus of "He Touched Me."

At 6 P.M. one summer evening, Art's life here on earth ended, and he stepped into the wonders of heaven. Thinking clearly and feeling well, no longer bewildered by dementia nor held back by an aging body, he's whole—and he's enjoying it!

> *He touched me,*
> *Oh, He touched me,*
> *And oh the joy that floods my soul.*
> *Something happened and now I know,*
> *He touched me and made me whole.*

*HE TOUCHED ME. Words and Music by William Gaither. Copyright © 1964 William J. Gaither, Inc. All rights controlled by Gaither Copyright Management. Used by permission.